Mycobacteriosis

Guest Editor

MIGUEL D. SAGGESE, DVM, MS, PhD

VETERINARY CLINICS OF NORTH AMERICA: EXOTIC ANIMAL PRACTICE

www.vetexotic.theclinics.com

Consulting Editor
AGNES E. RUPLEY, DVM, Dipl. ABVP–Avian

January 2012 • Volume 15 • Number 1

SAUNDERS an imprint of ELSEVIER, Inc.

W.B. SAUNDERS COMPANY
A Division of Elsevier Inc.

1600 John F. Kennedy Boulevard • Suite 1800 • Philadelphia, Pennsylvania 19103-2899

http://www.vetexotic.theclinics.com

VETERINARY CLINICS OF NORTH AMERICA: EXOTIC ANIMAL PRACTICE Volume 15, Number 1
January 2012 ISSN 1094-9194, ISBN-13: 978-1-4557-3951-6

Editor: John Vassallo; j.vassallo@elsevier.com
Developmental Editor: Teia Stone

Veterinary Clinics of North America: Exotic Animal Practice (ISSN 1094-9194) is published in January, May, and September by Elsevier, Inc., 360 Park Avenue South, New York, NY 10010-1710. Subscription prices are $229.00 per year for US individuals, $367.00 per year for US institutions, $117.00 per year for US students and residents, $273.00 per year for Canadian individuals, $433.00 per year for Canadian institutions, $308.00 per year for international individuals, $433.00 per year for international institutions and $150.00 per year for Canadian and foreign students/ residents. To receive student/resident rate, orders must be accompanied by name of affiliated institution, date of term, and the signature of program/residency coordinator on institution letterhead. Orders will be billed at individual rate until proof of status is received. Foreign air speed delivery is included in all *Clinics* subscription prices. All prices are subject to change without notice. **POSTMASTER:** Send address changes to *Veterinary Clinics of North America: Exotic Animal Practice*, Elsevier Health Sciences Division, Subscription Customer Service, 3251 Riverport Lane, Maryland Heights,MO63043. **Customer Service: Telephone: 1-800-654-2452** (U.S. and Canada); **1-314-447-8871** (outside U.S. and Canada). **Fax: 1-314-447-8029. E-mail: journalscustomerservice-usa@elsevier.com** (for print support); **journalsonlinesupport-usa@elsevier.com** (for online support).

Reprints. For copies of 100 or more of articles in this publication, please contact the Commercial Reprints Department, Elsevier Inc., 360 Park Avenue South, New York, New York 10010-1710. Tel.: (212)-633-3813; Fax: (212)-633-1935; E-mail: reprints@elsevier.com.

Veterinary Clinics of North America: Exotic Animal Practice is covered in *MEDLINE/PubMed (Index Medicus).*

Printed and bound by CPI Group (UK) Ltd, Croydon, CR0 4YY

Transferred to Digital Print 2012

Contributors

CONSULTING EDITOR

AGNES E. RUPLEY, DVM
Diplomate, American Board of Veterinary Practitioners–Avian Practice; Director and
Chief Veterinarian, All Pets Medical & Laser Surgical Center, College Station, Texas

GUEST EDITOR

MIGUEL D. SAGGESE, DVM, MS, PhD
Assistant Professor of Veterinary Microbiology and Avian/Wildlife Medicine, College of
Veterinary Medicine, Western University of Health Sciences, Pomona, California

AUTHORS

JENNIFER BUUR, DVM, PhD
Diplomate, American College of Veterinary Clinical Pharmacology; Assistant Professor
of Pharmacology, College of Veterinary Medicine, Western University of Health
Sciences, Pomona, California

BOB DAHLHAUSEN, DVM, MS
Veterinary Molecular Diagnostic, Inc, Milford, Ohio

J. JILL HEATLEY, DVM, MS
Diplomate, American Board of Veterinary Practitioners–Avian; Diplomate, American
College of Zoological Medicine; Associate Professor, Department of Small Animal
Clinical Sciences, Zoological Medicine Service, College of Veterinary Medicine and
Biomedical Sciences, Texas A&M University, College Station, Texas

FILIPE MARTINHO, DVM
Invited Teacher, Faculdade de Medicina Veterinária, Universidade Lusófona de
Humanidades e Tecnologias, Lisbon, Portugal

DIANE E. MCCLURE, DVM, PhD
Diplomate, American College of Laboratory Animal Medicine; Associate Professor of
Laboratory Animal Medicine, College of Veterinary Medicine, Western University of
Health Sciences, Pomona, California

MARK A. MITCHELL, DVM, MS, PhD
Diplomate, European College of Zoological Medicine–Herpetology; Professor,
Department of Veterinary Clinical Medicine, College of Veterinary Medicine, University of
Illinois, Urbana, Illinois

CHIARA PALMIERI, DVM, PhD
Diplomate, European College of Veterinary Pathologists; Faculty of Veterinary Medicine,
Veterinary Pathology Division, University of Teramo, Teramo, Italy

CHRISTAL POLLOCK, DVM
Diplomate, American Board of Veterinary Practitioners–Avian; Veterinary Consultant,
Lafeber Company, Cornell, Illinois

DRURY R. REAVILL, DVM
Diplomate, American Board of Veterinary Practitioners–Avian Practice; Diplomate, American College of Veterinary Pathologists; Zoo/Exotic Pathology Service, West Sacramento, California

MIGUEL D. SAGGESE, DVM, MS, PhD
Assistant Professor of Veterinary Microbiology and Avian/Wildlife Medicine, College of Veterinary Medicine, Western University of Health Sciences, Pomona, California

ROBERT E. SCHMIDT, DVM, PhD
Diplomate, American College of Veterinary Pathologists; Zoo/Exotic Pathology Service, West Sacramento, California

MARK D. SCHRENZEL, DVM, PhD
Diplomate, American College of Veterinary Pathologists; Hybla Valley Veterinary Hospital, Alexandria, Virginia

H.L. SHIVAPRASAD, BVSc, MS, PhD
Diplomate, American College of Poultry Veterinarians; Professor, Avian Pathology, California Animal Health and Food Safety Laboratory System–Tulare Branch, University of California, Davis, Tulare, California

DIEGO SOLER TOVAR, DVM, MS
College of Agricultural Sciences, Universidad de La Salle, Bogotá, Colombia

Contents

> The ecology of mycobacteria is shifting in accordance with environmental change and new patterns of interaction between wildlife, humans, and nondomestic animals. Infection of vertebrate hosts throughout the world is greater now than ever and includes a growing prevalence in free ranging and captive wild animals. Molecular epidemiologic studies using standardized methods with high discriminatory power are useful for tracking individual cases and outbreaks, identifying reservoirs, and describing patterns of transmission and are used with increasing frequency to characterize disease wildlife. This review describes current features of mycobacteriosis in wildlife species based on traditional descriptive studies and recent molecular applications.

> Mycobacteriosis is a serious disease across many animal species. Approximately more than 120 species are currently recognized in the genus Mycobacterium. This article describes the zoonotic potential of mycobacteria and mycobacteriosis in fish, amphibians, rodents, rabbits, and ferrets. It considers clinical signs; histology; molecular methods of identification, such as polymerase chain reaction and DNA sequencing; routes of infection; and disease progression. Studying the disease in animals may aid in understanding the pathogenesis of mycobacterial infections in humans and identify better therapy and preventative options such as vaccines.

> Avian mycobacteriosis is a disease that affects companion, captive exotic, wild, and domestic birds. The disease in birds is generally caused by *Mycobacterium avium* subsp *avium* but more than 10 other species of mycobacteria infect birds. Oral route of infection appears to be the primary mode of transmission. In some cases, the extensive involvement of the respiratory system suggests an airborne mode of transmission. Molecular diagnostic techniques have improved the ability to confirm the disease. Avian mycobacteriosis is an important

veterinary and economic risk in birds and mammals. Exposure of humans to infected birds may cause a zoonotic infection.

Treatment for avian mycobacteriosis is still in its infancy and based on extrapolations from human medicine. The optimum drug choice, dose, or length of treatment has yet to be determined for most exotic animal species. Treatment should include multiple drugs for extended periods of time with appropriate monitoring of both drug levels and overall animal health. Risk to owners and handlers needs to be minimized through appropriate identification of the species of mycobacteri causing disease. More research is necessary on the pharmacokinetics of these drugs in other animal species and antibiotic resistance. Currently, euthanasia remains the most common action in the face of active mycobacteriosis.

The term "mycobacteriosis" encompasses a variety of infectious diseases of animals caused by bacteria of the genus *Mycobacterium*, which are chronic and debilitating diseases. More than 35 *Mycobacterium* spp can cause mycobacteriosis. The wide range of possible clinical signs and physical exam findings can make the antemortem diagnosis inconsistent and challenging. Proper sample collection and test modality in relation to the state of the disease process are essential. Clinicians can determine a presumptive diagnosis of mycobacteriosis, but the definitive etiologic diagnosis of mycobacteriosis relies on the correct identification of the mycobacteria through microbiological and molecular diagnostic methods.

Spontaneous mycobacteriosis is rare in rabbits and rodents with the exception of the pygmy rabbit, and there are only a handful of reported cases involving other rodents. *Mycobacterium avium* complex was the most commonly identified organism in reports of spontaneous mycobacteriosis involving rabbits and rodents. The resistance of rabbits and rodents to mycobacterial disease has been useful in understanding the disease in humans and other animals. Preventing or controlling *Mycobacterium* sp transmission from wildlife to domestic animals will require collaboration between agriculture, wildlife, environmental, and political entities. Understanding the ecology and epidemiology of mycobacteria is needed for better worldwide management of tuberculosis.

Mycobacteriosis is an important disease worldwide. Although commonly associated with higher vertebrates, including humans, it has been reported in only a handful of reptile cases. The purpose of this article is to review the literature as it relates to mycobacteriosis in reptiles. Knowledge of the epidemiology of this disease can be useful to veterinarians working with these animals, especially when working on a diagnosis and making recommendations to clients regarding the need for case follow-up to rule in or rule out the potential presence of these pathogens in pet reptiles and best handling practices to minimize their exposure.

Amphibians are commonly kept in laboratory and zoological facilities and are becoming more frequent as pets. However, many amphibian species are declining in the wild owing to a variety of infectious and noninfectious diseases. This article reviews the current state of knowledge of mycobacteriosis in amphibian species, including pathogenesis, clinical signs, appropriate diagnostics, treatment options, and zoonotic potential and prevention. It is hoped this review will provide clinical veterinarians and scientists the tools they need to provide better care for amphibian species suffering mycobacteriosis, as well as serve to stimulate additional research into amphibians affected by mycobacterosis.

Mycobacteriosis is an important disease in the feral ferret (*Mustela putorius furo*) of New Zealand; elsewhere, reports of tuberculosis in the ferret are sporadic. Genus *Mycobacterium* consists of aerobic, non–spore-forming, gram-positive, nonmotile bacteria that characteristically feature a cell wall rich in mycolic acids and esters. The epidemiology of mycobacteriosis in the ferrets of New Zealand involves complex interactions between ferrets, possums, and livestock. Investigators have shown that the ferret is highly susceptible only to *Mycobacterium bovis* infection and is more resistant to infection by other *Mycobacterium* spp. The principal site of all mycobacterial infection in the ferret is the gastrointestinal tract.

RELATED INTEREST

Veterinary Clinics of North America: Small Animal Practice (Volume 41, Issue 6,
November 2011)
**Companion Animal Medicine: Evolving Infectious, Toxicological, and Parasitic
Diseases**
Sanjay Kapil, DVM, MS, PhD, *Guest Editor*

THE CLINICS ARE NOW AVAILABLE ONLINE!

Access your subscription at:
www.theclinics.com

Preface
Mycobacteriosis

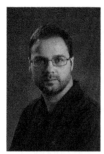

Miguel D. Saggese, DVM, MS, PhD
Guest Editor

It is an honor to be the guest editor of this special issue of the *Veterinary Clinics of North America: Exotic Animal Practice* fully devoted to mycobacterial infections in exotic pets and wildlife. They cause serious concerns among practitioners and exotic pet owners due to their potential zoonotic risk, challenging diagnosis, and lack of proven and effective treatment options. They are also a significant cause of mortality for several endangered wild avian and mammalian species being held at zoos and ongoing ex situ conservation efforts.

In recent years, a large body of new information and knowledge has been accumulated about mycobacterial infections in humans and, to a much lesser extent, exotic and wild animals. This information comes from a varied range of disciplines and experts working in this field, from molecular microbiologists, pathologists, and epidemiologists to exotic and wildlife veterinarians, physicians, and (let's not forget to mention them) graduate students from all around the world. Advances in molecular genetics, epidemiology, and diagnosis are providing new light into the precise identification of species and strains of mycobacteria affecting exotic pets and wildlife patients as well as into their relative zoonotic risk. Clinicians working on their cases in close relationship with pathologists and geneticists made significant contributions to our comprehension of the significance of the wide range of lesions and clinical presentations associated with these diseases. Etiological diagnosis can be achieved now in less than 24 hours through polymerase chain reaction and sequencing of specific genes. We have certainly made significant progress in the last decade. Nevertheless, we are still far from having a complete understanding of mycobacterial infection in the large and diverse number of species we work with every day. Current, scientific, and evidence-based information is key to providing effective advice to exotic pet owners or ex situ conservation programs managers. We have still too much to investigate and learn!

With this special issue, a large and diverse number of experts summarize the available information on mycobacteriosis in exotic pets and wildlife to provide a single

Vet Clin Exot Anim 15 (2012) ix–x
doi:10.1016/j.cvex.2011.12.002

reference source on a wide range of topics. At a same time, they provide new insights into areas of still-needed additional research, such as immune response, molecular epidemiology, treatment, genetic predispositions, and antimicrobial drug resistance, in mycobacterial isolates from exotic animals. Progress made during the last years in the fields of human tuberculosis and nontuberculous mycobacterial infections is certainly one of the most rapid and exciting areas of progress made in the world of infectious diseases. While important differences obviously exist between human and exotic pet mycobacterial infections, these advances could stimulate similar research in exotic pet patients and the species of mycobacteria affecting them. Then, with this special issue we hope to bring to the reader new and current information and at the same time identify existing gaps in our knowledge on mycobacterial diseases that will help us to make, perhaps in the next 10 years, significant new advances in this field through extensive research. Ultimately, this will help us improve the health of exotic pets and wildlife species with Mycobacteriosis.

I want to thank Dr Agnes Rupley for her encouragement and support for me to guest edit this special issue on mycobacteriosis. Special thanks to John Vassallo and all his staff at Elsevier for their oceans of patience, permanent help, and assistance during the elaboration and preparation of this issue. Finally, I am extremely indebted to the international panel of experts that contributed their knowledge and experiences. It has been a real pleasure to work with all of them and we hope that readers will find the information provided here useful and at the same time enjoy the reading of these articles as much as we did.

Miguel D. Saggese, DVM, MS, PhD
College of Veterinary Medicine
Western University of Health Sciences
309 East Second Street
Pomona, CA 91766, USA

E-mail address:
msaggese@westernu.edu

Molecular Epidemiology of Mycobacteriosis in Wildlife and Pet Animals

Mark D. Schrenzel, DVM, PhD, DACVP

KEYWORDS

- Molecular epidemiology • Mycobacteriosis • Wildlife
- Zoo animals

Mycobacterial infection of wildlife and nondomestic zoo and pet animals has been reported in hundreds of species and likely has the potential to occur in every vertebrate throughout the world. With the development of new molecular methods for detecting, naming, and characterizing microorganisms, the ecology of mycobacteria has rapidly advanced in all areas. In human medicine, polymerase chain reaction (PCR) assays are accepted diagnostic standards, replacing or complementing culture isolation and acid fast staining, while definitive criteria from the International Committee on Systematic Bacteriology for speciation and taxonomic placement of organisms are now derived primarily from multilocus DNA sequencing data rather than phenetic characteristics.[1–3] Progress in creating reliable fingerprints of bacteria has resolved members of the genus *Mycobacterium* into thousands of individual, traceable strains, and molecular epidemiology is now an essential component for addressing disease in all settings, from single patient case reports to regional epidemics.[4–6] In wildlife, applications of new technology have extended to studies in a wide range of nondomestic species. Over the past 10 years, there have been more than 150 reports of disease in nondomestic animals that use molecular analyses for speciation or strain-typing of the causative mycobacteria.

Mycobacteria have undergone extensive specialization with particular vertebrate hosts or specific environmental ecosystems over thousands of years while retaining the flexibility to occupy new niches by continually infecting different animals as primary pathogens or opportunists.[7] Wildlife, once sheltered by long standing ecological barriers, are emerging as novel targets of infection under growing anthropogenic pressures and, consequently, are driving critical aspects of mycobacterial disease dynamics as well as suffering the effects of infection by poorly adapted pathogens.[8] In this review, we provide update on mycobacterial ecology in wildlife, including captive nondomestic animals, from a molecular epidemiologic perspective,

The author has nothing to disclose.
Hybla Valley Veterinary Hospital, 7627 Richmond Highway, Alexandria, VA 22306, USA
E-mail address: mschrenzel@gmail.com

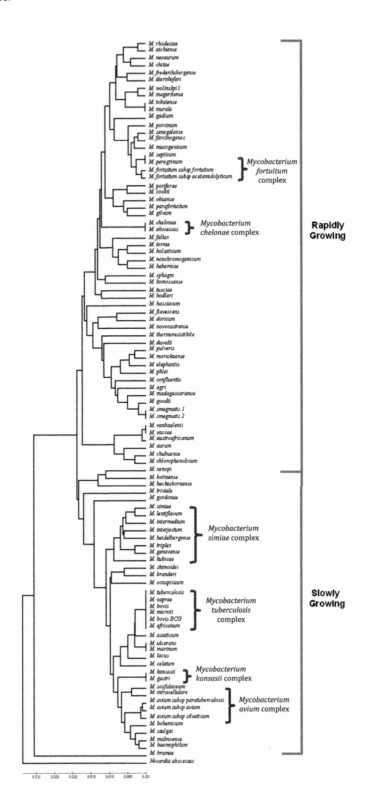

focusing on applications of recent technology and the agents that most profoundly impact veterinary and human medicine.

MOLECULAR EPIDEMIOLOGY

Molecular epidemiology uses methods for characterizing DNA or protein amino acid sequences in conjunction with epidemiologic analyses to describe the distribution and determinants of disease in defined populations. The term has generated some confusion, typically when data and inferences derived from molecular biomarkers, such as taxonomy, phylogeny, and population genetics, are used to describe disease with the exclusion of epidemiologic principles.[9] Conclusions about the origins and behavior of infectious agents denoted solely from molecular findings can be misleading. The use of genetic phylogenies, for example, to estimate ancestral origins, current day relatedness, and probable biologic effects of pathogens, such as potential host ranges or reservoirs, when used alone can obscure the real events occurring during disease transmission rather than providing useful insights. A distinction between microbial population genetics and microbial epidemiology is important for both scientists who design investigations and the clinicians who base decisions on the conclusions from these studies. Mycobacterial population genetics describes the breadth of genotypic variation, clonal origins of organisms, and how populations are organized in particular niches. It has benefitted greatly from advances in molecular biology and provided valuable insights into how mycobacteria interact with each other.[10,11] Used in conjunction with phenotypic traits, it has defined the genus *Mycobacterium* into more than 130 species and several subgroups of related bacteria, such as the *Mycobacterium tuberculosis* complex (MTC) and the *Mycobacterium avium* complex (MAC). The genetic organization of the genus is depicted in phylogenies or trees, which are useful for creating awareness of depth and evolution (**Fig. 1**). Molecular epidemiology uses the same molecular methods but applies them in a practical way to understand disease and has been especially useful for studying mycobacteria, which can be genetically and phenotypically monomorphic but exhibit widely differing host ranges and levels of disease expression. It determines causal relationships by integrating genetic findings with the basic tenets of epidemiology and newly evolving computational algorithms designed for molecular data, allowing the most appropriate medical intervention strategies and changes to animal husbandry or management practices.[10,11] This is particularly important in the study of wildlife disease where experimental methods, sample acquisition, and population definitions are difficult or impossible.

The 2 primary areas where molecular biology has joined epidemiology are diagnostics and strain-typing of pathogenic organisms:

PCR-based diagnostics of mycobacteria has received considerable support due to the difficulties of culture isolation and accuracy of acid-fast staining.[12] Challenges surrounding disruption of the resilient cell wall of mycobacteria for DNA extraction, the removal of PCR inhibitors from samples, and test sensitivity and specificity issues have been successfully addressed for many test protocols, and initial Food and Drug

←

Fig. 1. Relationship among *Mycobacterium* genus members shown with phylogenetic neighbor-joining tree using concatenated 16s rRNA and rpoB sequences calculated with Kimura's 2-parameter substitution model and rooted with *Nocardia abscessus*. Recognized complexes of organisms are shown with parentheses.

Administration–approved assays have been dramatically improved in recent years.[13,14] Now, approximately 90 of the 130 species in the genus have been linked to disease, many by PCR.[2,4,5,15] Fluorogenic real-time PCR platforms with the ability to detect multiple species in a single test and with sensitivities 10,000 times greater than conventional PCR and are used in veterinary diagnostics and research, including prospective and retrospective studies of wildlife mycobacteriosis.[16,17] In elephants, for example, PCR diagnostics is replacing culture detection for *M tuberculosis*,[18] and in a variety of species, formalin-fixed, paraffin-embedded tissues are being evaluated for mycobacterial infection with PCR.[17,19] For wildlife, zoo, and exotic animal veterinarian and scientists, consensus-based generic PCR assays able to detect and classify any type of mycobacteria in antemortem or postmortem samples are especially useful.[20,21]

Strain typing uses molecular techniques to create fingerprints of organisms. For mycobacteria, genomes of different species range from approximately 4.5 to 6.5 million base pairs and can include variable length repetitive elements and labile insertional sequences.[22–24] Numerous molecular typing methods that use DNA sequence data, PCR amplification, or enzymatic digestion of the genome or segments of the genome exist and have been customized to particular mycobacterial species. Each method has a different resolving power, and often, several techniques are combined in a study to identify the origins and patterns of spread of pathogens in epidemiologic analyses.[10,11] Genome sequencing offers the highest level resolution and is becoming more accessible as new-generation technology advances. PCR amplification of variable number tandem repeat (VNTR) elements and variable spacer elements (spoligotyping) has been standardized, resulting in global databases used to compare organisms from different locales.[11,25–27] Insertional sequences, because of their ability to move into and out of chromosomes, are often only present in some strains of mycobacteria and offer a rapid, economical typing method that can be used on clinical samples, like swabs, trunk washes, blood, or tissues, whereas most other methods require culture isolates. As mycobacteria are difficult to grow in vitro and sample collection is extremely variable in different settings, this feature is especially valuable in molecular epidemiology. Graphic data from insertional sequence, VNTR, and spoligotyping analyses are shown in **Fig. 2**.

To use information generated by molecular strain typing technology, new computational methods that incorporate detailed and complex genetic data into epidemiologic studies have been developed. These methods use different probability-based rules to estimate how quantitative genetic differences among strains translate into practical phenomena, such as origins and transmission patterns that can be used to prevent, contain, or eliminate infectious disease. Examples of some new, popular analyses are Structure, Structure-Neighbor clustering, and minimum spanning trees.[10,11] Structure is a Bayesian model method that groups individual microbial strains into populations based on the frequency probabilities of certain genetic signatures, usually single nucleotide polymorphisms.[28] Structure-Neighbor clustering is a similar, newly developed analysis that achieves more resolving power by adding another computation called nearest neighbor network clustering to the Structure analysis and is useful for characterizing mycobacteria with little genetic variation, such as members of MTC and *Mycobacterium leprae*, and minimum spanning trees are hierarchal clustering approaches that maximize inferences about disease by finding the minimum distance between related strains and placing these strains into groups. Often, minimum spanning trees use data dense typing methods of mycobacteria, such as VNTR fingerprints, which carry

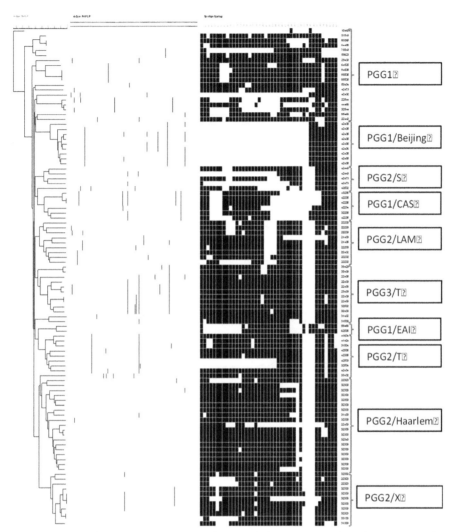

Fig. 2. Example of different strain typing data: *1*, phylogenetic tree based on copy number and genomic position of the mobile insertion site element IS6110; *2*, VNTR-based strain discrimination; *3*, spoligotype method of epidemiologically unrelated *M tuberculosis* isolates. The 3 strain typing methods demonstrate different visual fingerprints of unique strains and result in similar groupings that are also supported by Principal Genetic Group markers. (*Created and provided by* Dr Catherine Arnold, Applied and Functional Genomics Unit, Centre for Infections, Health Protection Agency, 61 Colindale Avenue, London NW9 5EQ, UK.)

the advantage of analyzing numerous loci as well as DNA segments that mutate at a higher rate than coding genes (**Fig. 3**).[10,11,29] All of these algorithms and similar methods use molecular information to create geographical maps or phylogeographies of pathogen strains that incorporate spatial and temporal data, allowing individual organisms to be traced to a potential reservoir and to visualize how they are moving within and between populations.[9–11,30]

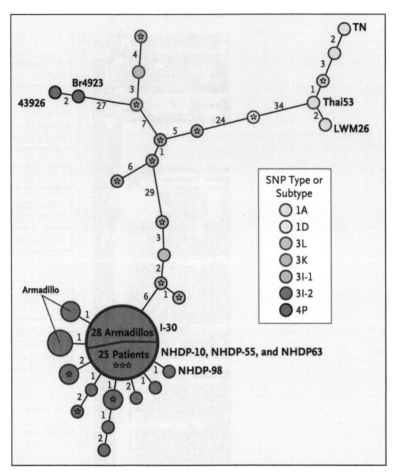

Fig. 3. Minimum-spanning phylogenetic tree of *Mycobacterium leprae* genotypes based on analysis of SNPs and VNTRs. Minimum-spanning-tree analysis was performed with the use of combined VNTR and SNP data from human and armadillo *M leprae* strains. Each circle represents a genotype (human unless marked as armadillo) based on the combined data, with the circle size directly proportional to the number of strains with the corresponding genotype. Numbers along the links between circles indicate the number of loci that differ between the genotypes on either side of the link. Three fully sequenced reference *M leprae* strains (TN, Thai53, and Br492322,29) are labeled, as are 2 other reference strains (LWM26 and 43926) of foreign origin. Samples from patients with a history of foreign residence are indicated with an asterisk (with 3 asterisks indicating three patients). The 114 polymorphisms investigated include 84 SNPs described previously, and 22 and 30 identified during our study; 10 VNTRs were also analyzed. The large circle illustrates the predominance of the 3I-2-v1 *M leprae* genotype in our study, with 25 patients and 28 armadillos having this identical genotype. (*Reprinted from* Truman RW, Singh P, Sharma R, et al. Probable zoonotic leprosy in the southern United States. N Engl J Med 2011;364:1626–33; with permission.)

Epidemiologic analyses are cornerstones of mycobacterial disease ecology that connect strain types with real events and remove many of the confounding factors, such as homoplasy (ie, common traits arising from convergent evolution) and horizontal gene transfer, that may occur in phylogenetic computations. For wildlife veterinarians, scientists, and conservation managers, awareness of the power of molecular epidemiology is important, particularly when allocating resources to address disease problems, as is knowledge of the potential limitations to these applications imposed by sample types. Innovations in molecular technology have created new possibilities for use of different kinds of samples but optimization of sample collection and archiving is essential when caring for rare, intractable animals. PCR diagnostics on paraffin-embedded materials and basic level strain typing on fluids or swabs with mixed microbial components are possible. However, ideal samples for mycobacterial molecular studies are pure culture clones isolated from clinical or postmortem samples. These provide a renewable source of DNA and can usually be easily acquired from diagnostic laboratories. For particular species, like M tuberculosis, sampling guidelines exist for different circumstances, but, in general, taking replicate samples from animals for microscopy (cytology or histology), culture, and molecular studies should be done when possible. For molecular studies, samples are best saved frozen, although dry storage on filter cards, lyophilization, dry storage in sterile vials, or immersion in buffers for nucleic acid preservation are viable alternatives.[31,32] Storage in ethyl alcohol at 70% or 100% is less desirable, although still useful, and formalin-fixation, especially at temperatures over 4°C, is the worst preservation method for molecular evaluations. General principles for sample handling and storage for molecular diagnostics of infectious agents have been outlined.[33–36]

Species are classified in the genus Mycobacterium using a variety of methods, such as complexes of genetically related organisms, pigmented and nonpigmented bacteria, slow and rapid growers, and tuberculous and nontuberculous mycobacteria. For wildlife, distinguishing between primary or strict pathogenic and opportunistic bacteria is important. Primary pathogenic mycobacteria have their primary niche within one or several hosts and result in variable levels of disease. Organisms can cause steadily progressive disease or be present within static microanatomic sites for years with little harm to the host and later become active, causing significant damage. Primary pathogenic mycobacteria can remain viable for variable periods in the environment but ultimately require living animal reservoirs to survive. Opportunists are mycobacteria whose lifestyle is adapted to living within environmental biotic communities but who can, in some situations, infect animal or human hosts and cause disease.[37] These bacteria lack maintenance hosts. In the past, the tuberculous mycobacteria were considered primary pathogens, while nontuberculous mycobacteria (NTM) (also known as mycobacteria other than tuberculosis [MOTT] or atypical mycobacteria) were viewed as opportunists.[37,38] However, this was chiefly an anthropocentric division, based on human medicine. In animals, it is best to maintain a conditional perception of organisms as established primary pathogens or probable opportunists when considering cases or outbreaks of disease with the realization that continuous levels of virulence and potentials to persist and be amplified in hosts exist in both groups and that molecular epidemiologic studies are essential for clarifying each organism's ecology.

PRIMARY PATHOGENS

Currently the second leading infectious cause of human mortality in the world, M tuberculosis is a global pandemic with a reservoir of approximately 2 billion infected people and is spreading into animals with increasing frequency.[39–42] For many years, M tuberculosis infection was recognized in zoo, laboratory, or exotic pet animals that had prolonged, close contact with people,[41,43] such as primates (rhesus macaques, cynomolgus monkeys, vervet monkey, great apes, and baboons), ungulates (African oryx, addax, black buck, bongo, camel, giraffe, buffalo, tapir, mountain goat, and rhinoceros), terrestrial carnivores (otter, polar bear), birds (parrot, macaw, and canary), and elephants.[43–48] Mycobacterium tuberculosis disease is now being found in free-ranging animals, such as mongooses and suricates in Africa, due to changes in the health, density, and travel habits of people.[40] In elephants, prevalence is increasing in some areas, and, currently, M tuberculosis is endemic in several Asian elephant populations.[49] Molecular epidemiologic studies using IS6110 restriction fragment length polymorphism (RFLP) analyses have documented elephant–human spread, confirming the longstanding supposition of zoonotic infection, and, conversely, there are extensive associative data to support transmission from people to elephants going back hundreds of years.[40,43,46,49–51] More importantly, recent molecular studies have demonstrated clonal elephant–elephant spread of M tuberculosis strains in multiple herds, suggesting that Asian elephants are likely maintenance hosts that can independently support infection and actively contribute to spillover–spillback dynamics.[49,50] Considering the number of people infected with M tuberculosis, the role of elephants in perpetuating human disease is insignificant. For elephants, however, animal–animal transmission with ongoing acquisitions from humans is a major threat to their survival. The seriousness of the problem is illustrated by recent findings that implicate tuberculosis as a major factor in the extinction of one of elephants' closest relatives, the mastodon.[52]

Mycobacterium bovis is closely related to M tuberculosis but is a primary pathogen of animals and has the broadest host range of any pathogenic mycobacterial species. The historical origin of M bovis predating animal domestication is not clear, but currently bovids, including domestic cattle, bison, and buffalo, are viewed as natural hosts.[51,53] Endemic infections of wildlife species having contact with these animals are considered reservoirs, and people as well as a numerous other animals— baboons, Colobus monkeys, macaques, gibbons, Patas monkeys, lemurs, chimpanzees, bears, leopards, lions, tigers, lynx, bobcats, hyenas, genets, raccoons, opossums, meerkats, foxes, llamas, alpacas, antelope, giraffes, sitatunga, topis, wildebeests, impalas, kudu, elands, yaks, Sika deer, axis deer, roe deer, muntjac, rabbits, camels, rhinoceroses, voles, moles, wood mice, brown rats, squirrels, ferrets, hyrax, oryx, and marine mammals—are accidental, dead end hosts that suffer from disease but do not consistently play a role in transmission.[26,48,51,53–59] Detection of M bovis infection or exposure with intradermal tuberculin skin testing or enzyme-linked immunosorbent assay has greatly decreased the incidence of infection in zoological parks and domestic animal facilities, but wildlife remain a continual source of infection in many parts of the world.[53,57,60]

Molecular epidemiologic studies defined the roles of wildlife species in spreading M bovis to cattle, humans, and other animals and have also been used to track disease outbreaks in free ranging and captive nondomestic animals. In the United Kingdom, factors causing the failure of M bovis eradication programs were clarified by strain typing data that identified Eurasian badgers (Meles meles) as a persistent source of infection for cattle and led to large-scale badger culling programs.[61,62] Culling efforts, however, unexpectedly resulted in an increased transmission to domestic cattle following a higher prevalence and morbidity in remaining badgers, and currently the Eurasian badger is a self-sustaining reservoir of M bovis in the United Kingdom and Ireland.[61–63] In France, by contrast, molecular studies using spoligotyping and VNTR analysis showed that badgers have no role in disease dynamics but rather wild boars (Sus scrofa) caused recurrent infection of cattle herds with a single stable strain of M bovis for more than 13 years.[64] In Spain, red deer (Cervus elaphus) and fallow deer (Dama dama) are also important hosts,[65] and many developed countries experience similar problems in their domestic animals and people due to wildlife reservoirs: in New Zealand, Brushtail possum (*Trichosurus vulpecula*)[63,66]; in South Africa, Buffalo (*Syncerus caffer*) and Kafue lechwe (*Kobus leche kafuensis*)[48,67]; in the United States, white-tailed deer (*Odocoileus virginianus*) and elk (*Cervus elaphus*)[63,68]; and, in Canada, wood bison (*Bison bison athabascae*) and elk[68] are maintenance hosts for *M bovis*. In Australia, although *M bovis* was eradicated from cattle, it remains endemic in feral pigs and feral Asian water buffalo (*Bubalus bubalis*).[54] A genome-based strain-typing study of more than 1000 isolates from over 30 countries recently showed that nearly all strains of *M bovis* in New Zealand, South Africa, North America, and Australia were derived from a single organism originating from Europe (chiefly the United Kingdom and Ireland), probably through international transport of infected cattle with secondary dispersal by wildlife reservoirs.[68] This strain, named clonal complex European 1, is now the most pervasive form of *M bovis* in the world and continues to have devastating effects on cattle, humans who have acquired infection from animals, and dozens of wildlife species on 3 continents.[68]

The dispersal and prevalence of *M bovis* in stable reservoirs make it a potential threat to all extant mammals, especially noncaptive animals.[48,53] In zoos, morbidity from *M bovis* infection still occurs but is no longer common due to better quarantine testing procedures.[56,57,69] In the United States and many developed countries, *M bovis* is a reportable pathogen. When disease is diagnosed in a controlled setting, government resources for strain typing are used to identify potential sources of infection, assess interspecies transmission events, and contain outbreaks.[56,69,70] In free ranging wildlife, *M bovis* is poorly regulated and continues to be problematic. Fatal infections steadily occur in threatened and endangered species, like cheetahs, lions, leopards, and black rhinoceroses.[71,72] *M bovis* strains often can be traced to large, mobile populations, like buffalo, lechwe, or greater kudu (*Tragelaphus strepsiceros*) in Africa or white-tailed deer, elk, wood bison, and American bison (*Bison bison*) in North America.[68,72,73] In southern Spain, bilateral transmission between regional domestic cattle and wild boars and deer resulted in penetration of *M bovis* throughout the Doñana National Park and exposure of naïve wildlife, including the endangered lynx.[63,74] These multihost systems facilitate survival of *M bovis* by lowering threshold population densities of reservoir species needed for disease persistence, and the free ranging behavior of hosts results in continual invasion of new ecosystems.[73] The result is constant pressure on atypical wildlife species and mortalities from chronic disease that promotes even greater dissemination.[68,75]

The MTC consists of organisms that are genetically very closely related, having arisen from a common ancestor, but exhibit different biologic effects and host tropisms. Members of the complex share 99.9% nucleotide identity and include eight species or ecotypes in addition to *M tuberculosis* and *M bovis* that can be discriminated using molecular strain typing tools.[76–78] Two species, *Mycobacterium africanum* and *Mycobacterium canettii*, are pathogens of people, although *M africanum* has been reported in hyrax (*Procavia capensis*) and milk from domestic cattle.[79,80] Another, *M bovis* bacillus Calmette-Guerin (BCG), is a vaccine strain of *M bovis*.[76] The remaining species occur at significant levels in nondomestic animals, all acting as primary pathogens. Like *M tuberculosis*, each has a proclivity for certain hosts but can on occasion infect other animals and cause disease. *Mycobacterium pinnipedii* targets pinnipeds (seals and sea lions) but has been recently been identified in a camel and Malayan tapirs. Spoligotyping of the isolates identified the source and probable routes of transmission among the animals at 2 zoological facilities, allowing measures to be taken to prevent future infections.[81] Infection has also been found in humans but is very rare.[82] The natural hosts of *Mycobacterium microti* are voles, wood mice, and shrews, but disease is periodically seen in humans, llamas, camels, badgers, and domestic cats.[83,84] *Mycobacterium caprae* is a pathogen of domestic goats and occurs sporadically in domestic sheep, wild boar, red deer, and humans.[85–87] The oryx bacillus is a distinct ecotype in the complex originally isolated from oryx in Saudia Arabia and the Netherlands but has emerged in the past several years in buffalo in South Africa.[88,89] The final member, the dassie bacillus, has thus far only been confirmed in rock hyrax.[76,90]

Collectively, the members of MTC share features of being primary or strict pathogens with little genetic diversity. A bottleneck event followed by co-speciation of the ten members with different hosts that began approximately 20,000 years ago is a widely accepted explanation for the genetic relatedness but different host preferences of the members.[78] *M bovis* differs from other species in having an extremely broad host range and clearly represents the biggest threat to most mammalian wildlife.[53,68] Molecular epidemiologic studies coupled with preventative strategies, such as segregating domestic and nondomestic animals, more extensive testing of animals being moved, and BCG vaccination of wildlife, offer hope for reducing disease from all members of the MTC.[68,91]

M leprae causes disease chiefly in people and armadillos. Rarely, other animals (chimpanzees, mangabeys, and cynomolgus macaques) are infected.[92–94] Like members of the MTC, *M leprae* is a strict pathogen but is more monomorphic, having single nucleotide polymorphisms (SNPs) every 28,000 base pairs compared to *M tuberculosis*, which has polymorphisms every 200 base pairs.[95] The genetic homogeneity of *M leprae*, along with the inability to grow it in culture, the presence of numerous pseudogenes, and a clinical latency period of 2 to 3 years, make it a unique and challenging agent to study. Despite these obstacles, high resolution VNTR and SNP analyses have been useful in tracing movement of strains and have identified a new "American" type organism whose presence strongly supports transmission of *M leprae* from free ranging armadillo populations to people in the southwestern United States (**Fig. 3**).[94] Although leprosy infection is now curable with antibiotics, the disease often leaves debilitating and disfiguring lesions in skin and nerves, and the zoonotic risk of armadillo populations with endemic *M leprae* is creating concern in local human populations.[94,96]

M leprae also causes disease in armadillos consisting of granulomatous inflammation, especially in nerves, lymph nodes, and the nasal cavity.[97] The cooler body temperature (89°C) of armadillos and features of the immune system are well suited for the leprae bacillus, and intraspecies transmission occurs readily among armadillos via direct contact with nasal or oral excretions and, probably, soil organisms derived from infected animals.[96,98] Prevalence rates in some populations are 15%. However, it should be noted that New World armadillos acquired *M leprae* from humans during early European expeditions and are not a natural host.[94]

M avium subsp *paratuberculosis* is a major health threat to captive wildlife throughout the world and also has extensive reservoirs in free-ranging animals. The organism was named based on its genetic similarity to *M avium* subsp *avium* but differs by acting as a primary pathogen of ruminants.[99,100] PCR-based speciation methods targeting the insertional element, IS900, or other *M avium* subsp *paratuberculosis*–specific genes, such as F57, have improved detection in biologic and environmental samples.[101] Among nonruminants, *M avium* subsp *paratuberculosis* has now been described in tissues from rabbits, foxes, stoats, weasels, badgers, wood mice, Norway rats, European brown hares, jackdaws, rooks, wild boars, wallabies, kangaroos, humans, and crows and in feces from raccoons, armadillos, a giraffe, an opossum, and rhesus macaques.[19,100,102–105] Detailed studies on wild rabbits indicate that they are important reservoirs of *M avium* subsp *paratuberculosis*.[106,107] The extent to which other wildlife affects the ecology of *M avium* subsp *paratuberculosis* needs to be clarified. Most carnivores are likely dead end hosts with no impact on disease dynamics.[105] However, it is evident that *M avium* subsp *paratuberculosis* has a broad host range and the potential for dispersal and persistence through diverse pathways.[100]

Ruminants and camelids throughout the world continue to experience losses from *M avium* subsp *paratuberculosis*.[99,107,108] In zoos, cryptic reservoirs exist in the form of clinically normal ruminants, and new infections occur despite investment in routine herd screening, quarantine testing, and culling of suspect individuals.[99] In the wild, numerous free-ranging species, such as deer, bighorn sheep, elk, buffalo, and bison, suffer from disease.[99,100,102] The stability of infection among these populations has not been reliably established but is likely to be substantial due to the chronicity of disease, probable existence of nonruminant reservoirs or accidental hosts, and ongoing exposure from domestic animals.

Molecular epidemiologic studies have been valuable for tracking spread of *M avium* subsp *paratuberculosis* and understanding strain-associated virulence and infectivity.[99] Data from captive and wild animals have divided most isolates into distinct, host-associated genotypes, such as sheep (type I), cattle (type II), bird and bison strains.[99,105,109] These studies have been useful for investigating transmission patterns in different settings and indicate that extensive interspecies strain sharing occurs with even strongly host-associated organisms able to infect new targets in their environment.[99,105,110] As contact patterns between people, domestic animals, and wildlife continue to shift, the ecological distribution of *M avium* subsp *paratuberculosis* is expected to grow. Invasion of *M avium* subsp *paratuberculosis* into nondomestic animal populations, such as free ranging nilgai in India and wild guanacos in Chile, and into new environmental niches, including drinking water and meat in the United States, are increasing.[110–113]

Mycobacterium lepraemurium causes leprosy in its natural hosts (mice and rats) and in an aberrant host, domestic cats, and is considered a strict pathogen by most, although little is known about its biology.[92] It is serologically and genetically related to *M avium* subsp *avium* and appears to be unculturable.[114] Many descriptions of *M lepraemurium* concern its experimental use in rodents as a model of human leprosy, and no molecular strain typing studies have been reported. Consequently, the prevalence, burden, and extent of interspecies transmission, other than that occurring with cats, remain unknown.[92,115]

Mycobacterium marinum and *Mycobacterium ulcerans* are closely related to the MTC, particularly *M tuberculosis*, but exist to a large extent in the environment and may be considered as primary or opportunistic pathogens depending on host and situational factors.[116] *M marinum* causes mycobacteriosis in numerous fish and amphibian species and has also been found in reptiles, hedgehogs, manatees, and humans.[117,118] It is also the most commonly identified cause of mycobacterial disease in reptiles.[119] In fish, most disease outbreaks have occurred in aquaculture or aquarium facilities, but wild populations have been found with prevalence rates as high as 75%.[120] Strain typing methods with strong discriminatory power have failed to identify strain-specific patterns of virulence or geographical associations for *M marinum*, and the organism appears to be a genetically rich mixture of mobile aquatic saprophytes with pathogenic potential in both vertebrates and invertebrates.[121–125] *Mycobacterium ulcerans* is the closest relative of *M marinum* but differs in one key aspect. Both species excrete a myolactone polyketide that is an ulcer-causing cytotoxin, but *M marinum* also has the region of difference 1 (RD1) chromosomal segment containing the *esat-6* and *cfp-1* virulence genes that are essential for intracellular survival in phagolysosomes.[126] RD1 is present in *M tuberculosis*, *M kansasii*, *M szulgai*, and *M riyadhense* but not *M ulcerans*. Consequently, *M ulcerans* is an extracellular pathogen that infects a wide diversity of hosts, including possums, black rats, koalas, fish, snails, and numerous species of insects.[127–129] Unlike *M marinum*, which is largely free-living in water, *M ulcerans* appears to survive primarily within animals. Insects are a large reservoir and are probably vectors for mammalian species.[130,131] In mosquitoes, PCR studies have shown that the expression of the myolactone is essential for *M ulcerans* to colonize mouth parts and be efficiently transmitted to animals during feeding bites.[130] VNTR strain analyses in possums demonstrated that both ringtail and brushtail possums are important reservoirs of *M ulcerans* and transmit infections to people in addition to suffering from ulcerative disease themselves.[128]

OPPORTUNISTIC PATHOGENS

The distinction between primary or strict pathogens and opportunists is most tenuous when the role of the environment in transmission is considered. An environmental source of infection in which organisms remain viable in a suspended state and an environmental reservoir where organisms live and replicate are descriptors used to define fundamental aspects of epidemiology for different mycobacteria. However, crossover between these areas may occur and, for most species, the dynamics underlying development of disease in different hosts is complex. Many of the primary pathogens are viable outside their hosts for substantial periods. *M bovis* can remain infective for up to 88 days in soil, 55 days in water and hay, and 43 days on corn.[132] *M leprae* occurs at a much higher density in soil samples adjacent to areas with endemic infection and can remain viable in soil and possibly water for long periods.[98] *M avium* subsp *paratuberculosis*, which can survive for more than 1 year in the environment, also replicates within environmental amoeba.[133,134]

Less is known about mycobacterial opportunists. By definition, all can live and reproduce outside hosts. Some species, such as *M avium* subsp *avium*, exhibit wide ranges of behavior, including extracellular replication in environmental biome communities, intracellular survival, replication, and dispersal in water-born Acanthamoeba, and infectivity for a broad range of vertebrate hosts.[133,135,136] Even for *M avium* subsp *avium*, however, strain-related differences in virulence, seeding of environmental niches following amplification in animals, and consequences of adaptive traits conferring host infectivity on environmental survival are poorly understood.[133,135]

Mycobacterium genavense is a significant avian pathogen and also causes disease in immunocompromised people. It has been found by PCR in a kangaroo, squirrel, dwarf rabbit, lemur, and 2 ferrets but most often occurs in psittacine and passerine birds and HIV-positive people.[19,136–139] Despite being a well-recognized and persistent cause of disease, little is known about its natural habitats and reservoirs. As a nontuberculous *Mycobacterium*, it is often viewed as an environmental organism and has been found in water supplies.[138,140,141] However, molecular strain typing methods for *M genavense* consist only of basic MLST, and the genome has not yet been characterized.[142] Observational data from numerous reports of human cases suggest that infections originate from both environmental and avian sources.[136,138,140] In birds, the majority of reported illness has been in captive animals, and the extent of disease in free ranging, wild species is not known.[136,139]

The MAC is a group of related organisms that is variably defined in the context of clinical medicine, science, and taxonomy to include approximately 5 subspecies, all of which differ significantly in their biology.[114] Among the members, *Mycobacterium intracellulare* is genetically easily distinguished from the others and is an important cause of pneumonia, lymphadenitis, and arthritis in immunocompetent people.[143] In wildlife, it is a recognized disease of birds and has been on occasion reported in baboons, ferrets, and marsupials (numbats, wallabies, and Tasmanian devils), which are particularly vulnerable to mycobacteria in general.[75,144] Domestic swine also regularly acquire *M intracellulare* and develop lymphadenitis, while infection in cattle is usually self-limiting.[144,145] Advanced strain typing methods were developed to allow precise tracking of *M intracellulare* isolates and have been used in 2 major hosts—people and swine. In both cases, environmental sources of infection were predominant. Water, in particular, was a frequent source of organisms and appears to be a special niche for *M intracellulare* as it is able to establish high density colonies in aqueous biofilms.[114,146,147] Further analyses are needed to establish transmission routes that exist in birds.[114,148] *M avium* subsp *avium* infection also occurs sporadically in a number of mammalian wildlife species and is the most common cause of avian mycobacteriosis. Like *M intracellulare*, it occurs in domestic swine throughout the world but is not common in cattle.[114,144,148–151] In people, disease is typically associated with immunocompromise or debilitation.[114] Molecular epidemiologic studies support primary environmental sources of infection in humans, birds, and swine with a lesser role of direct transmission between hosts but need to be extended to fully understand how and why disease develops.[114,136,152,153] Searches for molecular markers of virulence, such as IS910, will be important for understanding the complexities of opportunistic infection in all animals.[154] Strain typing and whole genome studies comparing isolates found in diseased humans and birds have not been done but will, likewise, be essential for identifying situational, host, and bacteria-related factors involved in producing disease.

M avium subsp *silvaticum* and *M avium* subsp *hominissuis* comprise the remaining members of MAC. *M avium* subsp *silvaticum* causes disease in wood pigeons and remains a point of controversy regarding its distinction from *M avium* subsp *avium*. Among wildlife, it appears to be limited to infrequent infections in birds.[114] *M avium* subsp *hominissuis* is a genetically diverse group of strains, similar to *M avium* subsp *avium*, that opportunistically infect swine and humans. VNTR and mycobacterial interspersed repetitive units (MIRU) fingerprints and minimum spanning tree analyses show that most infections derive from environmental reservoirs.[155–157] Infection of nondomestic animals is rare with 1 report in a parrot.[158]

Numerous other NTM occur in wildlife. Most are infrequent pathogens; however, several species have been linked to disease with some regularity. *Mycobacterium fortuitum* and *M chelonae* comprise the *M fortuitum* complex and, along with *M marinum*, are notable opportunistic pathogens of fish, reptiles, and, less often, amphibians and may even be considered as primary pathogens in some situations.[17,116–119,159] Strain typing methods for the complex show that the group is composed of genetically diverse organisms with a strong environmental reservoir, similar to the MAC.[160–162] *Mycobacterium kansasii* infection has been reported in deer, squirrel monkeys, and birds but, more so, is recognized as a cause of disease in people. Specific strain-associated virulence pattern have been useful in tracing sources of *M kansasii* infections in humans.[163] For other mycobacteria, molecular epidemiologic methods and application in studies are rare but with increased awareness of their importance will likely grow. Mycobacterial species linked to disease are summarized in **Table 1**.

Table 1
Primary and opportunistic pathogens of wildlife, nondomestic animals, humans, and exotic pet animals

Small carnivores/omnivores include domestic ferrets; birds include pet birds; suids, and ruminants comprise only feral species. Mycobacteria species shown in bold are considered primary pathogens for the corresponding hosts, and those listed below are most often viewed as opportunistic pathogens.

Primates	**M tuberculosis, M leprae, M africanum**
	M bovis, M simiae, M avium subsp *paratuberculosis,*
	   M intracellulare, M gordonae, M avium subsp *avium,*
	   M kansasii, M scofulaceum, M arctoides

Humans	**M tuberculosis, M leprae, M africanum**
	M bovis, M simiae, M avium subsp *paratuberculosis,*
	   M intracellulare, M avium subsp *avium, M kansasii,*
	   M scrofulaceum, M arctoides, M gordonae, M ulcerans,
	   M marinum, M abscessus, M haemophilum, M celatum,
	   M margeritense, Mlentiflavum, M septicum, M massiliense,
	   M chelonae, M smegmatis, M asiaticum, M genavense,
	   M microti, M bolletii, M arosiense, M noviomagense,
	   M malmoense, M chimaera, M lacus, M heckehornense,
	   M avium subsp *hominissuis, M cannetti, M conspicuum,*
	   M branderi, M kyorinense, M gastri, M shimoidei, M szulgai,
	   M bohemicum, M peregrinum, M riyadhense, M vaccae,
	   M fortuitum, M pinnipedi

Ruminants	**M bovis, M avium** subsp **paratuberculosis** *M caprae, M tuberculosis, M africanum, M aurum, M intracellulare,* *M celatum, M xenopi, M asiaticum, M vaccae, M fortuitum*
Camelids	**M bovis, M avium** subsp **paratuberculosis** *M microti, M kansasii*
Small Carnivores/Omnivores	**M bovis, M ulcerans, M leprae** *M tuberculosis, M avium* subsp *paratuberculosis, M microti,* *M fortuitum, M celatum, M avium* subsp *avium, M genavense*
Rodents	**M microti, M lepraemurium** *M fortuitum, M vaccae, M bovis, M avium* subsp *avium,* *M avium* subsp *paratuberculosis*
Suids	**M bovis** *M avium* subsp *hominissuis, M avium* subsp *avium,* *M intracellulare, M bohemicum, M szulgai*

Birds	*M genavense, M avium* subsp *avium, M intracellulare,*
	   M intermedium, M peregrinum, M terrae,
	   M avium subsp *paratuberculosis, M avium* subsp *hominissuis,*
	   M trivial, M fortuitum, M diernhoferi, M chelonae,
	   M smegmatis, M flavescens, M scrofulaceum

Marine Mammals	**M pinnipedii** *M marinum, M bovis, M margaritense, M chelonae*

Fish	*M marinum, M chelonae, M fortuitum, M ulcerans,*
	   M pseudoshottsii, M salmoniphilum, M insubricum,
	   M stomatepiae, M peregrinum, M abscessus,
	   M haemophilum, M shottsii, M montefiorense, M neoarum,
	   M simiae, M scofulaceum, M gordonae, M chesapeaki,
	   M septicum, M avium subsp *avium, M triplex*

Reptiles	*M chelonae, M szulgai, M marinum, M kansasii,* *M haemophilum, M intracellulare*

(continued on next page)

Table 1 (continued)	
Amphibians	*M marinum, M liflandii*
Domestic Horses	*M bovis, M ulcerans, M avium* subsp *hominissuis, M avium* subsp *avium, M smegmatis, M terrae, M avium* subsp *paratuberculosis*
Domestic Dogs	*M tuberculosis, M bovis, M avium* subsp *avium, M avium* subsp *hominissuis, M chelonae, M flavescens, M fortuitum, M goodie, M microti, M kansasii, M smegmatis*
Domestic Cats	*M lepraemurium, M bovis, M fortuitum, M microti, M avium* subsp *avium, M ulcerans, M xenopi, M abscessus, M massiliense, M alvei, M avium* subsp *paratuberculosis, M simiae, M smegmatis, M terrae, M genavense, M thermoresistibile, M mucogenicum, M szulgai, M septicum*

SUMMARY

Mycobacteria comprise the most numerous and diverse primary and opportunistic pathogenic bacteria of animals and humans and continue to rapidly evolve as global ecosystems change. Determinants of pathogenicity have been investigated for decades through in vivo and in vitro studies and retrospective analyses of naturally occurring cases, leading to significant improvements in health. Yet, due to continual changes in host-pathogen dynamics and the natural complexity of factors dictating the outcome of infections, mycobacteriosis continues to be a leading cause of illness. Advances in molecular epidemiology, including technologic breakthroughs, standardization of investigative methods, and communal databases, have begun to dramatically change perspectives and therapeutics for disease among clinicians and scientists. Utilization of PCR for diagnostics will continue to be especially important in veterinary medicine as most mycobacteria are difficult to isolate by culture. Accessibility to widely used strain typing methods from individual cases or disease outbreaks provided to practitioners by granting agencies and government supported research centers throughout the world is, likewise, paramount for mitigating future morbidity.

Mycobacterial infections in humans continue to rise, and disease in wildlife, nondomestic animals, and exotic pet animals is growing in parallel. By using current diagnostic methods and providing case materials to research centers for molecular epidemiologic analyses, veterinarians can significantly improve animal and human health.

ACKNOWLEDGMENTS

The author thanks Madoka Sumitani for editorial assistance and Dr Barry Hall and Dr Catherine Arnold for their contributions.

REFERENCES

1. Devulder G, Pérouse de Montclos M, Flandrois JP. A multigene approach to phylogenetic analysis using the genus Mycobacterium as a model. Int J Syst Evol Microbiol 2005;55(Pt 1):293–302.
2. Tortoli E. Impact of genotypic studies on mycobacterial taxonomy: the new mycobacteria of the 1990s. Clin Microbiol Rev 2003;16:319–54.

3. Clarridge JE 3rd. Impact of 16S rRNA gene sequence analysis for identification of bacteria on clinical microbiology and infectious diseases. Clin Microbiol Rev 2004; 17:840–62.
4. Rastogi N, Legrand E, Sola C. The mycobacteria: an introduction to nomenclature and pathogenesis. Rev Sci Tech 2001;20:21–54.
5. Behr MA, Falkinham JO 3rd. Molecular epidemiology of nontuberculous mycobacteria. Fut Microbiol 2009;4:1009–20.
6. Driscoll JR. Spoligotyping for molecular epidemiology of the *Mycobacterium tuberculosis* complex. Methods Mol Biol 2009;551:117–28.
7. Smith NH, Gordon SV, de la Rua-Domenech R, et al. Bottlenecks and broomsticks: the molecular evolution of *Mycobacterium bovis*. Nat Rev Microbiol 2006;4:670–81.
8. Pavlin BI, Schloegel LM, Daszak P. Risk of importing zoonotic diseases through wildlife trade, United States. Emerg Infect Dis 2009;15:1721–6.
9. Foxman B, Riley L. Molecular epidemiology: focus on infection. Am J Epidemiol 2001;153:1135–41.
10. Salipante SJ, Hall BG. Towards the molecular epidemiology of *Mycobacterium leprae*: strategies, successes, and shortcomings. Infect Genet Evol 2011;11: 1505–13.
11. Hall BG, Salipante SJ. Molecular epidemiology of *Mycobacterium leprae* as determined by structure-neighbor clustering. J Clin Microbiol 2010;48:1997–2008.
12. Hofmann-Thiel S, Turaev L, Hoffmann H. Evaluation of the hyplex TBC PCR test for detection of *Mycobacterium tuberculosis* complex in clinical samples. BMC Microbiol 2010;10:95.
13. Leung ET, Zheng L, Wong RY, et al. Rapid and simultaneous detection of *Mycobacterium tuberculosis* complex and Beijing/W genotype in sputum by an optimized DNA extraction protocol and a novel multiplex real-time PCR. J Clin Microbiol 2011;49:2509–15.
14. Mehrotra R, Metz P, Kohlhepp S. Comparison of in-house polymerase chain reaction method with the Roche Amplicor technique for detection of *Mycobacterium tuberculosis* in cytological specimens. Diagn Cytopathol 2002;26:262–5.
15. Tortoli E, Baruzzo S, Heijdra Y, et al. *Mycobacterium insubricum* sp. nov. Int J Syst Evol Microbiol 2009;59:1518–23.
16. Sweeney FP, Courtenay O, Hibberd V, et al. Environmental monitoring of *Mycobacterium bovis* in badger feces and badger sett soil by real-time PCR, as confirmed by immunofluorescence, immunocapture, and cultivation. Appl Environ Microbiol 2007; 73:7471–3.
17. Zerihun MA, Hjortaas MJ, Falk K, et al. Immunohistochemical and Taqman real-time PCR detection of mycobacterial infections in fish. J Fish Dis 2011;34:235–46.
18. Kay MK, Linke L, Triantis J, et al. Evaluation of DNA extraction techniques for detecting *Mycobacterium tuberculosis* complex organisms in Asian elephant trunk wash samples. J Clin Microbiol 2011;49:618–23.
19. Cleland PC, Lehmann DR, Phillips PH, et al. A survey to detect the presence of *Mycobacterium avium* subspecies *paratuberculosis* in Kangaroo Island macropods. Vet Microbiol 2010;145:339–46.
20. Kox LF, van Leeuwen J, Knijper S, et al. PCR assay based on DNA coding for 16S rRNA for detection and identification of mycobacteria in clinical samples. J Clin Microbiol 1995;33:3225–33.
21. Wu X, Zhang J, Liang J, et al. Comparison of three methods for rapid identification of mycobacterial clinical isolates to the species level. J Clin Microbiol 2007;45:1898–903.

22. Stinear TP, Seemann T, Harrison PF, et al. Insights from the complete genome sequence of Mycobacterium marinum on the evolution of *Mycobacterium tuberculosis*. Genome Res 2008;18:729–41.
23. Zhang ZY, Sun ZQ, Wang ZL, et al. Complete genome of a novel clinical isolated non-tuberculous mycobacterium strain JDM601. J Bacteriol 2011;193:4300–1.
24. Li L, Bannantine JP, Zhang Q, et al. The complete genome sequence of *Mycobacterium avium subspecies paratuberculosis*. Proc Natl Acad Sci U S A 2005;102:12344–9.
25. Brudey K, Driscoll, JR, Rigouts L, et al. *Mycobacterium tuberculosis* complex genetic diversity: mining the fourth international spoligotyping database (SpolDB4) for classification, population genetics and epidemiology. BMC Microbiol 2006;6:23.
26. Duarte EL, Domingos M, Amado A, et al. Spoligotype diversity of *Mycobacterium bovis* and *Mycobacterium caprae* animal isolates. Vet Microbiol 2008;130:415–21.
27. Barandiaran S, Martínez Vivot M, Moras EV, et al. *Mycobacterium bovis* in Swine: spoligotyping of isolates from Argentina. Vet Med Int 2011;id979647.
28. Pritchard JK, Stephens M, Rosenberg NA, et al. Association mapping in structured populations. Am J Hum Genet 2000;67:170–81.
29. Kang HY, Wada T, Iwamoto T, Phylogeographical particularity of the *Mycobacterium tuberculosis* Beijing family in South Korea based on international comparison with surrounding countries. J Med Microbiol 2010;59:1191–7.
30. Thierry S, Wang D, Arné P, et al. Multiple-locus variable-number tandem repeat analysis for molecular typing of *Aspergillus fumigatus*. BMC Microbiol 2010;10:315.
31. Aye KS, Matsuoka M, Kai M, et al. FTA card utility for PCR detection of *Mycobacterium leprae*. Jpn J Infect Dis 2011;64:246–8.
32. Owens CB, Szalanski AL. Filter paper for preservation, storage, and distribution of insect and pathogen DNA samples. J Med Entomol 2005;42:709–11.
33. Derion T. Considerations for the planning and conduct of reproducibility studies of in vitro diagnostic tests for infectious agents. Biotechnol Annu Rev 2003;9:249–58.
34. Grody W, Nakamura R, Strom C, et al, editors. Molecular diagnostics: techniques and applications for the clinical laboratory. New York: Academic Press; 2010.
35. Bruns D, Ashwood E, Burtis C, editors. Fundamentals of molecular diagnostics. New York: Saunders/Elsevier; 2007.
36. Leonard D, Bagg A, editors. Molecular pathology in clinical practice. London: Springer; 2007.
37. Petrini B. Non-tuberculous mycobacterial infections. Scand J Infect Dis 2006;38: 246–55.
38. Kankya C, Muwonge A, Djønne B, et al. Isolation of non-tuberculous mycobacteria from pastoral ecosystems of Uganda: public health significance. BMC Public Health 2011;11:320.
39. Sandhu GK. Tuberculosis: current situation, challenges and overview of its control programs in India. J Glob Infect Dis 2011;3:143–50.
40. Alexander KA, Pleydell E, Williams MC, et al. *Mycobacterium tuberculosis*: an emerging disease of free-ranging wildlife. Emerg Infect Dis 2001;8:598–601.
41. Michalak K, Austin C, Diesel S, et al. *Mycobacterium tuberculosis* infection as a zoonotic disease: transmission between humans and elephants. Emerg Infect Dis 1998;4:283–7.
42. Malik AN, Godfrey-Faussett P. Effects of genetic variability of *Mycobacterium tuberculosis* strains on the presentation of disease. Lancet Infect Dis 2005;5: 174–83.
43. Montali RJ, Mikota SK, Cheng LI. *Mycobacterium tuberculosis* in zoo and wildlife species. Rev Sci Tech 2001;20:291–303.

44. Fourie PB, Odendaal MW. *Mycobacterium tuberculosis* in a closed colony of baboons (Papio ursinus). Lab Anim 1983;17:125–8.
45. Schmidt V, Schneider S, Schlomer J, et al. Transmission of tuberculosis between men and pet birds: a case report. Avian Pathol 2008;37:589–92.
46. Lewerin SS, Olsson SL, Eld K, et al. Outbreak of *Mycobacterium tuberculosis* infection among captive Asian elephants in a Swedish zoo. Vet Rec 2005;156:171–5.
47. Une Y, Mori T. Tuberculosis as a zoonosis from a veterinary perspective. Comp Immunol Microbiol Infect Dis 2007;30:415–25.
48. Kaneene JB, Miller R, de Kantor IN, et al. Tuberculosis in wild animals. Int J Tuberc Lung Dis 2010;14:1508–12.
49. Mikota SK, Maslow JN. Tuberculosis at the human-animal interface: an emerging disease of elephants. Tuberculosis (Edinb) 2011;91:208–11.
50. Payeur JB, Jarnagin JL, Marquardt JG, et al. Mycobacterial isolations in captive elephants in the United States. Ann N Y Acad Sci 2002;969:256–8.
51. O'Reilly LM, Daborn CJ. The epidemiology of *Mycobacterium bovis* infections in animals and man: a review. Tuberc Lung Dis 1995;76(Suppl 1):1–46.
52. Rothschild BM, Laub R. Hyperdisease in the late Pleistocene: validation of an early 20th century hypothesis. Naturwissenschaften 2006;93:557–64.
53. Corner LA, Murphy D, Gormley E. *Mycobacterium bovis* infection in the Eurasian badger (Meles meles): the disease, pathogenesis, epidemiology and control. J Comp Pathol 2011;144:1–24.
54. Corner LA. The role of wild animal populations in the epidemiology of tuberculosis in domestic animals: how to assess the risk. Vet Microbiol 2006;112:303–12.
55. Renner M, Bartholomew WR. Mycobacteriologic data from two outbreaks of bovine tuberculosis in nonhuman primates. Am Rev Respir Dis 1974;109:11–6.
56. Stetter MD, Mikota SK, Gutter AF, et al. Epizootic of *Mycobacterium bovis* in a zoologic park. J Am Vet Med Assoc 1995;207:1618–21.
57. Mann PC, Bush M, Janssen DL, Clinicopathologic correlations of tuberculosis in large zoo mammals. J Am Vet Med Assoc 1981;179:1123–9.
58. Wilson P, Weavers E, West B, et al. *Mycobacterium bovis* infection in primates in Dublin Zoo: epidemiological aspects and implications for management. Lab Anim 1984;18:383–7.
59. Mathews F, Macdonald DW, Taylor GM, et al. Bovine tuberculosis (*Mycobacterium bovis*) in British farmland wildlife: the importance to agriculture. Proc Biol Sci 2006;273:357–65.
60. Adams LG. In vivo and in vitro diagnosis of *Mycobacterium bovis* infection. Rev Sci Tech 2001;20:304–24.
61. Vial F, Donnelly CA. Localized reactive badger culling increases risk of bovine tuberculosis in nearby cattle herds. Biol Lett 2011. [Epub ahead of print].
62. Gormley E, Costello E. Tuberculosis and badgers: new approaches to diagnosis and control. J Appl Microbiol 2003;94:80S–6S.
63. Naranjo V, Gortazar C, Vicente J, et al. Evidence of the role of European wild boar as a reservoir of *Mycobacterium tuberculosis* complex. Vet Microbiol 2008;127:1–9.
64. Zanella G, Durand B, Hars J, *Mycobacterium bovis* in wildlife in France. J Wildl Dis 2008;44:99–108.
65. Romero B, Aranaz A, Sandoval A, et al. Persistence and molecular evolution of *Mycobacterium bovis* population from cattle and wildlife in Doñana National Park revealed by genotype variation. Vet Microbiol 2008;132:87–95.
66. Palmer MV. Tuberculosis: a reemerging disease at the interface of domestic animals and wildlife. Curr Top Microbiol Immunol 2007;315:195–215.

67. de Garine-Wichatitsky M, Caron A, Gomo C, et al. Bovine tuberculosis in buffaloes, Southern Africa. Emerg Infect Dis 2010;16:884–5.
68. Smith NH, Berg S, Dale J, et al. European 1: A globally important clonal complex of *Mycobacterium bovis*. Infect Genet Evol 2011;11:1340–51.
69. Thorel MF, Karoui C, Varnerot A, et al. Isolation of *Mycobacterium bovis* from baboons, leopards and a sea-lion. Vet Res 1998;29:207–12.
70. Twomey DF, Crawshaw TR, Anscombe JE, et al. Assessment of antemortem tests used in the control of an outbreak of tuberculosis in llamas (*Lama glama*). Vet Rec 2011;167:475–80.
71. Espie IW, Hlokwe TM, Gey van Pittius NC, et al. Pulmonary infection due to *Mycobacterium bovis* in a black rhinoceros (*Diceros bicornis minor*) in South Africa. J Wildl Dis 2009;45:1187–93.
72. Michel AL, Coetzee ML, Keet DF, et al. Molecular epidemiology of *Mycobacterium bovis* isolates from free-ranging wildlife in South African game reserves. Vet Microbiol 2009;133:335–43.
73. Renwick AR, White PC, Bengis RG. Bovine tuberculosis in southern African wildlife: a multi-species host-pathogen system. Epidemiol Infect 2007;135:529–40.
74. Gortazar C, Torres MJ, Acevedo P, et al. Fine-tuning the space, time, and host distribution of mycobacteria in wildlife. BMC Microbiol 2011;11:27.
75. Buddle BM, Young LJ. Immunobiology of mycobacterial infections in marsupials. Dev Comp Immunol 2000;24:517–29.
76. Vasconcellos SE, Huard RC, Niemann S, et al. Distinct genotypic profiles of the two major clades of *Mycobacterium africanum*. BMC Infect Dis 2010;10:80.
77. Cousins DV, Bastida R, Cataldi A, et al. Tuberculosis in seals caused by a novel member of the Mycobacterium tuberculosis complex: *Mycobacterium pinnipedii sp. nov.* Int J Syst Evol Microbiol 2003;53:1305–14.
78. Brosch R, Gordon SV, Marmiesse M, et al. A new evolutionary scenario for the *Mycobacterium tuberculosis* complex. Proc Natl Acad Sci U S A 2002;99:3684–9.
79. Cadmus SI, Yakubu MK, Magaji AA, et al. *Mycobacterium bovis*, but also *M africanum* present in raw milk of pastoral cattle in north-central Nigeria. Trop Anim Health Prod 2010;42:1047–8.
80. Gudan A, Artuković B, Cvetnić Z, et al. Disseminated tuberculosis in hyrax (Procavia capensis) caused by *Mycobacterium africanum*. J Zoo Wildl Med 2008;39:386–91.
81. Moser I, Prodinger WM, Hotzel H, et al. *Mycobacterium pinnipedii*: transmission from South American sea lion (*Otaria byronia*) to Bactrian camel (*Camelus bactrianus bactrianus*) and Malayan tapirs (*Tapirus indicus*). Vet Microbiol 2008;127:399–406.
82. Kiers A, Klarenbeek A, Mendelts B, et al. Transmission of *Mycobacterium pinnipedii* to humans in a zoo with marine mammals. Int J Tuberc Lung Dis 2008;12:1469–73.
83. Zanolari P, Robert N, Lyashchenko KP, et al. Tuberculosis caused by *Mycobacterium microti* in South American camelids. J Vet Intern Med 2009;23:1266–72.
84. Xavier Emmanuel F, Seagar AL, et al. Human and animal infections with *Mycobacterium microti*, Scotland. Emerg Infect Dis 2007;13:1924–7.
85. Rodríguez E, Sánchez LP, Pérez S, et al. Human tuberculosis due to *Mycobacterium bovis* and *M caprae* in Spain, 2004–2007. Int J Tuberc Lung Dis 2009;13:1536–41.
86. Cunha MV, Matos F, Canto A, et al. Implications and challenges of tuberculosis in wildlife ungulates in Portugal: a molecular epidemiology perspective. Res Vet Sci 2011. [Epub ahead of print].
87. Muñoz Mendoza M, Juan LD, Menéndez S, et al. Tuberculosis due to *Mycobacterium bovis* and *Mycobacterium caprae* in sheep. Vet J 2011. [Epub ahead of print].

88. Huard RC, Fabre M, de Haas P, et al. Novel genetic polymorphisms that further delineate the phylogeny of the *Mycobacterium tuberculosis* complex. J Bacteriol 2006;188:4271–87.

89. van Helden PD, Parsons SD, Gey van Pittius NC. 'Emerging' mycobacteria in South Africa. J S Afr Vet Assoc 2009;80:210–4.

90. Parsons S, Smith SG, Martins Q, et al. Pulmonary infection due to the dassie bacillus (*Mycobacterium tuberculosis* complex sp.) in a free-living dassie (rock hyrax-*Procavia capensis*) from South Africa.Tuberculosis (Edinb) 2008;88:80–3.

91. Buddle BM, Wedlock DN, Denis M, et al. Update on vaccination of cattle and wildlife populations against tuberculosis. Vet Microbiol 2011;151:14–22.

92. Rojas-Espinosa O, Løvik M *Mycobacterium leprae* and *Mycobacterium lepraemurium* infections in domestic and wild animals. Rev Sci Tech 2001;20:219–51.

93. Loughry WJ, Truman RW, McDonough CM, et al. Is leprosy spreading among nine-banded armadillos in the southeastern United States? J Wildl Dis 2009;45: 144–52.

94. Truman RW, Singh P, Sharma R, et al. Probable zoonotic leprosy in the southern United States. N Engl J Med 2011;364:1626–33.

95. Achtman M. Evolution, population structure, and phylogeography of genetically monomorphic bacterial pathogens. Annu Rev Microbiol 2008;62:53–70.

96. Scollard DM, Adams LB, Gillis TP, et al. The continuing challenges of leprosy. Clin Microbiol Rev 2006;19:338–81.

97. Walsh GP, Meyers WM, Binford CH. Naturally acquired leprosy in the nine-banded armadillo: a decade of experience 1975–1985. J Leukoc Biol 1986;40:645–56.

98. Lavania M, Katoch K, Katoch VM, et al. Detection of viable *Mycobacterium leprae* in soil samples: insights into possible sources of transmission of leprosy. Infect Genet Evol 2008;8:627–31.

99. Manning EJ. *Mycobacterium avium subspecies paratuberculosis*: a review of current knowledge. J Zoo Wildl Med 2001;32:293–304.

100. Corn JL, Manning EJ, Sreevatsan S, et al. Isolation of *Mycobacterium avium subsp paratuberculosis* from free-ranging birds and mammals on livestock premises. Appl Environ Microbiol 2005;71:6963–7.

101. Sidoti F, Banche G, Astegiano S, et al. Validation and standardization of IS900 and F57 real-time quantitative PCR assays for the specific detection and quantification of *Mycobacterium avium subsp paratuberculosis*. Can J Microbiol 2011;57:347–54.

102. Singh SV, Singh AV, Singh PK, et al. Molecular identification and characterization of *Mycobacterium avium subspecies paratuberculosis* in free living non-human primate (Rhesus macaques) from North India. Comp Immunol Microbiol Infect Dis 2011;34: 267–71.

103. Beard PM, Daniels MJ, Henderson D, et al. Paratuberculosis infection of nonruminant wildlife in Scotland. J Clin Microbiol 2001;39:1517–21.

104. Alvarez J, De Juan L, Briones V, et al. *Mycobacterium avium* subspecies *paratuberculosis* in fallow deer and wild boar in Spain. Vet Rec 2005;156:212–3.

105. Stevenson K, Alvarez J, Bakker D, et al. Occurrence of *Mycobacterium avium subspecies paratuberculosis* across host species and European countries with evidence for transmission between wildlife and domestic ruminants. BMC Microbiol 2009;9:212.

106. Davidson RS, Marion G, White PC, et al. Use of host population reduction to control wildlife infection: rabbits and paratuberculosis. Epidemiol Infect.2009;137:131–8.

107. Salgado M, Manning EJ, Monti G, et al. European Hares in Chile: A Different Lagomorph Reservoir for *Mycobacterium avium* subsp *paratuberculosis*? J Wildl Dis 2011;47:734–8.

108. Alharbi KB, Al-Swailem A, Al-Dubaib MA, et al. Pathology and molecular diagnosis of paratuberculosis of camels. Trop Anim Health Prod 2011. [Epub ahead of print].

109. Semret M, Turenne CY, de Haas P, et al. Differentiating host-associated variants of *Mycobacterium avium* by PCR for detection of large sequence polymorphisms. J Clin Microbiol 2006;44:881–7.

110. Kumar S, Singh SV, Singh AV, et al. Wildlife (Boselaphus tragocamelus)-small ruminant (goat and sheep) interface in the transmission of "Bison type" genotype of *Mycobacterium avium subspecies paratuberculosis* in India. Comp Immunol Microbiol Infect Dis 2010;33:145–59.

111. Whittington RJ, Begg DJ, de Silva K, et al. Comparative immunological and microbiological aspects of paratuberculosis as a model mycobacterial infection. Vet Immunol Immunopathol 2011. [Epub ahead of print].

112. Gill CO, Saucier L, Meadus WJ. *Mycobacterium avium* subsp *paratuberculosis* in dairy products, meat, and drinking water. J Food Prot 2011;74:480–99.

113. Beumer A, King D, Donohue M, et al. Detection of *Mycobacterium avium subsp paratuberculosis* in drinking water and biofilms by quantitative PCR. Appl Environ Microbiol 2010;76:7367–70.

114. Turenne CY, Wallace R Jr, Behr MA. *Mycobacterium avium* in the postgenomic era. Clin Microbiol Rev 2007;20:205–29.

115. Rojas-Espinosa O, Becerril-Villanueva E, Wek-Rodríguez K, et al. Palsy of the rear limbs in *Mycobacterium lepraemurium*-infected mice results from bone damage and not from nerve involvement. Clin Exp Immunol 2005;140:436–42.

116. Stamm LM, Brown EJ. *Mycobacterium marinum*: the generalization and specialization of a pathogenic mycobacterium. Microbes Infect 2004;6:1418–28.

117. Sato T, Shibuya H, Ohba S, et al. Mycobacteriosis in two captive Florida manatees (*Trichechus manatus latirostris*). J Zoo Wildl Med 2003;34:184–8.

118. Bercovier H, Vincent V. Mycobacterial infections in domestic and wild animals due to *Mycobacterium marinum*, *M fortuitum*, *M chelonae*, *M porcinum*, *M farcinogenes*, *M smegmatis*, *M scrofulaceum*, *M xenopi*, *M kansasii*, *M simiae* and *M genavense*. Rev Sci Tech 2001;20:265–90.

119. Murray M, Waliszewski NT, Garner MM, et al. Sepsis and disseminated intravascular coagulation in an eastern spiny softshell turtle (*Apalone spinifera spinifera*) with acute mycobacteriosis. J Zoo Wildl Med 2009;40:572–5.

120. Kaattari IM, Rhodes MW, Kaattari SL, et al. The evolving story of *Mycobacterium tuberculosis* clade members detected in fish. J Fish Dis 2006;29:509–20.

121. Sun G, Chen C, Li J, et al. Discriminatory potential of a novel set of Variable Number of Tandem Repeats for genotyping *Mycobacterium marinum*. Vet Microbiol 2011; 152(1-2):200–4.

122. Stragier P, Ablordey A, Meyers WM, et al. Genotyping *Mycobacterium ulcerans* and *Mycobacterium marinum* by using mycobacterial interspersed repetitive units. J Bacteriol 2005;187:1639–47.

123. De la Torre C, Vega A, Carracedo A, et al. Identification of *Mycobacterium marinum* in sea-urchin granulomas. Br J Dermatol 2001;145:114–6.

124. Jernigan JA, Farr BM. Incubation period and sources of exposure for cutaneous *Mycobacterium marinum* infection: case report and review of the literature. Clin Infect Dis 2000;31:439–43.

125. Blackwell V. *Mycobacterium marinum* infections. Curr Opin Infect Dis 1999;12: 181–4.

126. van Ingen J, de Zwaan R, Dekhuijzen R, et al. Region of difference 1 in nontuberculous Mycobacterium species adds a phylogenetic and taxonomical character. J Bacteriol 2009;191:5865–7.

127. Portaels F, Chemlal K, Elsen P, et al. *Mycobacterium ulcerans* in wild animals. Rev Sci Tech 2001;20:252–64.
128. Fyfe JA, Lavender CJ, Handasyde KA, et al. A major role for mammals in the ecology of *Mycobacterium ulcerans*. PLoS Negl Trop Dis 2010;4:e791.
129. Durnez L, Suykerbuyk P, Nicolas V, et al. Terrestrial small mammals as reservoirs of *Mycobacterium ulcerans* in benin. Appl Environ Microbiol 2010;76:4574–7.
130. Tobias NJ, Seemann T, Pidot SJ, et al. Mycolactone gene expression is controlled by strong SigA-like promoters with utility in studies of *Mycobacterium ulcerans* and buruli ulcer. PLoS Negl Trop Dis 2009;3:e553.
131. Marsollier L, Brodin P, Jackson M, et al. Impact of *Mycobacterium ulcerans* biofilm on transmissibility to ecological niches and Buruli ulcer pathogenesis. PLoS Pathog 2007;3:e62.
132. Fine AE, Bolin CA, Gardiner JC, et al. A Study of the Persistence of *Mycobacterium bovis* in the Environment under Natural Weather Conditions in Michigan, USA. Vet Med Int 2011:ui765430.
133. Mura M, Bull TJ, Evans H, et al. Replication and long-term persistence of bovine and human strains of *Mycobacterium avium* subsp *paratuberculosis* within Acanthamoeba polyphaga. Appl Environ Microbiol 2006;72:854–9.
134. Pribylova R, Slana I, Kaevska M, et al. Soil and plant contamination with *Mycobacterium avium* subsp *paratuberculosis* after exposure to naturally contaminated mouflon feces. Curr Microbiol 2011;62:1405–10.
135. Cirillo JD, Falkow S, Tompkins LS, et al. Interaction of *Mycobacterium avium* with environmental amoebae enhances virulence. Infect Immun 1997;65:3759–67.
136. Tell LA, Woods L, Cromie RL. Mycobacteriosis in birds. Rev Sci Tech 2001;20:180–203.
137. Ludwig E, Reischl U, Janik D, et al. Granulomatous pneumonia caused by *Mycobacterium genavense* in a dwarf rabbit (*Oryctolagus cuniculus*). Vet Pathol 2009;46:1000–2.
138. Hillebrand-Haverkort ME, Kolk AH, Kox LF, et al. Generalized *Mycobacterium genavense* infection in HIV-infected patients: detection of the mycobacterium in hospital tap water. Scand J Infect Dis 1999;31:63–8.
139. Theuss T, Aupperle H, Eulenberger K, et al. Disseminated infection with *Mycobacterium genavense* in a grizzled giant squirrel (Ratufa macroura) associated with the isolation of an unknown Mycobacterium. J Comp Pathol 2010;143:195–8.
140. Manarolla G, Liandris E, Pisoni G, et al. Avian mycobacteriosis in companion birds: 20-year survey. Vet Microbiol 2009;133:323–7.
141. Portaels F, Realini L, Bauwens L, et al. Mycobacteriosis caused by *Mycobacterium genavense* in birds kept in a zoo: 11-year survey. J Clin Microbiol 1996;34:319–23.
142. Leclerc MC, Haddad N, Moreau R, et al. Molecular characterization of environmental mycobacterium strains by PCR-restriction fragment length polymorphism of hsp65 and by sequencing of hsp65, and of 16S and ITS1 rDNA. Res Microbiol 2000;151:629–38.
143. Dauchy FA, Dégrange S, Charron A, et al. Variable-number tandem-repeat markers for typing *Mycobacterium intracellulare* strains isolated in humans. BMC Microbiol 2010;10:93.
144. Thorel MF, Huchzermeyer HF, Michel AL. *Mycobacterium avium* and *Mycobacterium intracellulare* infection in mammals. Rev Sci Tech 2001;20:204–18.
145. Lara GH, Ribeiro MG, Leite CQ, et al. Occurrence of *Mycobacterium spp.* and other pathogens in lymph nodes of slaughtered swine and wild boars (Sus scrofa). Res Vet Sci 2011;90:185–8.

146. Ramasoota P, Chansiripornchai N, Källenius G, et al. Comparison of *Mycobacterium avium* complex (MAC) strains from pigs and humans in Sweden by random amplified polymorphic DNA (RAPD) using standardized reagents. Vet Microbiol 2001;78:251–9.
147. Alvarez J, García IG, Aranaz A, et al. Genetic diversity of *Mycobacterium avium* isolates recovered from clinical samples and from the environment: molecular characterization for diagnostic purposes. J Clin Microbiol 2008;46:1246–51.
148. Napier JE, Hinrichs SH, Lampen F, et al. An outbreak of avian mycobacteriosis caused by *Mycobacterium intracellulare* in little blue penguins (Eudyptula minor). J Zoo Wildl Med.2009;40:680–6.
149. Glawischnig W, Steineck T, Spergser J. Infections caused by *Mycobacterium avium subspecies avium, hominissuis*, and *paratuberculosis* in free-ranging red deer (Cervus elaphus hippelaphus) in Austria, 2001–2004. J Wildl Dis 2006;42:724–31.
150. Stepanova H, Pavlova B, Stromerova N, et al. Cell-mediated immune response in swine infected with *Mycobacterium avium* subsp *avium*. Vet Immunol Immunopathol 2011;142:107–12.
151. Harrenstien LA, Finnegan MV, Woodford NL, et al. *Mycobacterium avium* in pygmy rabbits (Brachylagus idahoensis): 28 cases. J Zoo Wildl Med 2006;37:498–512.
152. Kauppinen J, Hintikka E, Iivanainen E, et al. PCR-based typing of *Mycobacterium avium* isolates in an epidemic among farmed lesser white-fronted geese (*Anser erythropus*). Vet Microbiol 2001;81:41–50.
153. Thegerström J, Marklund BI, Hoffner S, et al. *Mycobacterium avium* with the bird type IS1245 RFLP profile is commonly found in wild and domestic animals, but rarely in humans. Scand J Infect Dis 2005;37:15–20.
154. Dvorska L, Bull TJ, Bartos M, et al. A standardised restriction fragment length polymorphism (RFLP) method for typing *Mycobacterium avium* isolates links IS901 with virulence for birds. J Microbiol Methods 2003;55:11–27.
155. Bruijnesteijn van Coppenraet LE, de Haas PE, et al. Lymphadenitis in children is caused by *Mycobacterium avium hominissuis* and not related to "bird tuberculosis." Eur J Clin Microbiol Infect Dis 2008;27:293–9.
156. Pate M, Kušar D, Zolnir-Dovč M, et al. MIRU-VNTR typing of Mycobacterium avium in animals and humans: heterogeneity of *Mycobacterium avium subsp. hominissuis* versus homogeneity of *Mycobacterium avium subsp. avium* strains. Res Vet Sci 2010;91(3):376–81.
157. Iwamoto T, Nakajima C, Nishiuchi Y, et al. Genetic diversity of *Mycobacterium avium subsphominissuis* strains isolated from humans, pigs, and human living environment. Infect Genet Evol 2011. [Epub ahead of print].
158. Shitaye EJ, Grymova V, Grym M, et al. *Mycobacterium avium subsp hominissuis* infection in a pet parrot. Emerg Infect Dis 2009;15:617–9.
159. Fremont-Rahl JJ, Ek C, Williamson HR, et al. *Mycobacterium liflandii* outbreak in a research colony of *Xenopus (Silurana) tropicalis* frogs. Vet Pathol 2011;48:856–67.
160. Esteban J, Molleja A, Cabria F, et al. SDS-PAGE for identification of species belonging to the *Mycobacterium fortuitum* complex. Clin Microbiol Infect 2003;9:327–31.
161. Sampaio JL, Chimara E, Ferrazoli L, et al. Application of four molecular typing methods for analysis of *Mycobacterium fortuitum* group strains causing post-mammaplasty infections. Clin Microbiol Infect 2006;12:142–9.
162. Ortiz A, Esteban J, Zamora N. Molecular identification by random amplified polymorphic DNA analysis of a pseudo-outbreak of *Mycobacterium fortuitum* due to cross-contamination of clinical samples. J Med Microbiol 2007;56:871–2.
163. Iwamoto T, Saito H. Comparative study of two typing methods, hsp65 PRA and ITS sequencing, revealed a possible evolutionary link between *Mycobacterium kansasii* type I and II isolates. FEMS Microbiol Lett 2006;254:129–33.

Mycobacterial Lesions in Fish, Amphibians, Reptiles, Rodents, Lagomorphs, and Ferrets with Reference to Animal Models

Drury R. Reavill, DVM, Dipl. ABVP (Avian Practice), Dipl. ACVP*,
Robert E. Schmidt, DVM, PhD, Dipl. ACVP

KEYWORDS

- Fish • Amphibians • Reptiles • Rodents • Lagomorphs
- Ferrets • Mycobacteria

Mycobacteriosis is a serious disease across many animal species and has been described in the scientific literature since the 1880s. Approximately more than 120 species are currently recognized in the genus *Mycobacterium*.[1] Mycobacteria differ greatly in their ecology, from the obligate pathogen *Mycobacterium tuberculosis*, which is a leading cause of human mortality worldwide, to saprophytic soil residents such as *M terrae*.[2]

A number of classification schemes have been used to characterize this bacterium. Historically, Mycobacteria were divided in three groups for the purposes of diagnosis: (1) the *M tuberculosis* complex (MTC), which includes *M tuberculosis*, *M bovis*, *M africanum*, *M microti*, *M canetti*, *M caprae*, *M pinnipedii*, and for some authors, *M marinum* and *M ulcerans*; (2) *M leprae*, which causes Hansen's disease or leprosy; and (3) mycobacteria other than the *M tuberculosis* complex (MOTT) or nontuberculous mycobacteria (NTM), comprising *M avium*, *M intracellulare*, *M marinum*, *M ulcerans*, *M lepraemurium*, and atypical mycobacteria.[3–5]

The Runyon classification (introduced by Ernest Runyon in 1959)[6] of nontuberculous mycobacteria is based on the rate of growth, production of yellow pigment, and whether this pigment was produced in the dark or only after exposure to light. Fast growers require less than 7 days to produce colonies on solid agar, whereas slow growers may require weeks to months. Both fast- and slow-growing species may be

---

The authors have nothing to disclose.
Zoo/Exotic Pathology Service, 2825 KOVR Drive, West Sacramento, CA 95605, USA
* Corresponding author. 7647 Wachtel Way, Citrus Heights, CA 95610.
E-mail address: DReavill@zooexotic.com

Vet Clin Exot Anim 15 (2012) 25–40
doi:10.1016/j.cvex.2011.10.001
1094-9194/12/$ – see front matter © 2012 Elsevier Inc. All rights reserved.

nonpigmented, photochromogenic (form pigment in response to light), or scotochromogenic (form pigment in the absence of light).[2,5]

The status of *M marinum* and *M ulcerans* is currently under examination. They are both closely related to *M tuberculosis*; however, are not considered part of the MTC group. *M marinum* cannot be distinguished from *M ulcerans* by ribosomal gene sequencing because they are so closely related that taxonomists argue if these two microorganisms really represent a single species. *M ulcerans* appears to have recently evolved from *M marinum* by reductive evolution and plasmid acquisition. Currently molecular evaluation is greatly expanding what is known about relatedness of all these organisms and assisting in rapid identification.[5,7–10] Both *M marinum* and *M ulcerans* are faster growing than *M tuberculosis* and more closely related than other mycobacterial species, which makes them useful models for studying the pathogenesis of *M tuberculosis*.[4]

Diagnosis of mycobacteriosis requires detection of acid-fast bacteria in exudates, fine-needle aspirates, or tissue biopsy specimens; culture; or detection using polymerase chain reaction (PCR) techniques. Isolation by culture and biochemical analysis has been the traditional method used in the identification of mycobacteria. However, mycobacteria tend to be slow-growing organisms (compared to other bacteria) and biochemical analysis is not only time consuming but also does not definitively distinguish between various species. Molecular methods (PCR and DNA sequencing) are proving to be a rapid and common method of identification. The list of recognized mycobacterial isolates and species continues to grow, reflecting the advancement and acceptance of molecular characterization of species.

ZOONOTIC POTENTIAL OF MYCOBACTERIA

Many of the mycobacterial species isolated from animals have a zoonotic potential.[11] This has been well documented with *M marinum* and this organism is classically associated with dermatologic lesions in aquarists.[12–14] *M abscessus*, *M fortuitum*, and *M chelonae* are also responsible for skin and soft tissue infection in humans.[14]

The zoonotic potential of *M genavense* and *M haemophilum*, mycobacterial pathogens requiring special conditions for laboratory culture, have also been described.[15] *M genavense* is an atypical, difficult to grow bacterium that has been isolated from organ transplant recipients or from patients concurrently infected with human immunodeficiency virus. It is the most commonly recognized cause of mycobacterial infections in pet birds.[5] Human infections by *M haemophilum* frequently are associated with septic arthritis, osteomyelitis, and pneumonia, generally restricted to immunocompromised patients.[12,15] Zebrafish appear to be particularly vulnerable to *M haemophilum*.

M kansasii, a member of the atypical group of mycobacteria, has been reported to produce chronic pulmonary disease resembling tuberculosis and chronic granulomatous dermatitis in humans.[16–18] It has been recognized as an infection in a Chinese soft shell turtle (*Pelodiscus sinensis*) and from the aqueous environment of ornamental fish tanks.[17,19]

Buruli ulcer caused by *M ulcerans*, a previously uncommon emerging disease, has recently been reported as the second most frequent mycobacterial disease in humans after tuberculosis in some countries. This bacterium is found in association with rivers, swamps, and wetlands. The mode of transmission remains unclear, although vectors such as aquatic insects, adult mosquitoes, or other biting arthropods are suspected. It has been isolated from fish and an Indian flap-shelled turtle (*Lissemys punctata punctata*).[20,21]

FISH MYCOBACTERIOSIS

All freshwater, brackish water, and saltwater fish are susceptible to mycobacteria and there are extensive reviews of these infections in the literature.[2,8,14,22–30] Mycobacteriosis is one of the most common chronic infections of fish, both wild and commercial.[26,31] The published incidence ranges from 15% in some wild fish populations to 40% and even reaching 100% in closed systems.[24–27,32] Fish submissions examined at the authors' laboratory identified mycobacterial infections in 4.3% of cases.

The mycobacteria most commonly reported in fish include *M marinum*, *M fortuitum*, and *M chelonae*.[9,27,29] Other common isolates from fish are *M neoaurum*, *M peregrinum*, *M gordonae*, *M haemophilum*, *M simiae*, *M scrofulaceum*, *M montefiorense*, *M poriferae*, *M shottsii*, *M pseudoshottsii*, *M chesapeaki* (isolated from wild striped bass, *Moroxone saxatilis*), and *M ulcerans*.[8–10,26] Granulomatous skin lesions in moray eels yielded *M triplex*.[8] From four lined seahorses (*Hippocampus erectus*) the inflammatory exudates in the gas bladders were due to *M poriferae*. The inflammation was histiocytic in both the kidney and gas bladder, but typical granulomas were not identified.[33] From case material at the authors' service, the identified species were *M gordonae*, *M chelonae*, *M marinum*, and *M haemophilum*. The most common visceral organs affected were the spleen, kidney, and liver.

The routes of infection are by ingestion of contaminated food or from a carrier or subclinically infected fish. In the 1950s, *M chelonae* infections in Pacific salmon were an important economic problem. The disease incidence was greatly reduced when pasteurized salmon viscera and other fish products were used as foodstuffs.[31] It has been documented to be spread from infected fish via shedding through the gastrointestinal tract.[34] Lesions in the skin and gills can be responsible for dissemination of the organisms in the environment. In some viviparous fish, it can be transmitted transovarially.[22,23,35]

In general, mycobacteriosis presents as a chronic wasting disease lasting from months to years.[14] Clinical signs include emaciation, sunken abdomen, external ulcerations, fin rot, deformities of the spinal column, exophthalmia, changes in normal coloration (faded in aquarium fish and bright colors in salmonids), and lifting of scales.[26,36]

A rare, acute, fulminating form has been described.[5,36–38] This experimentally induced form is characterized by a systemic mycobacterial infection, with severe peritonitis, tissue necrosis, celomic cavity fluid accumulation, edema, skin ulceration, fin erosions, and a short survival time.[5,38]

The chronic form is a disseminated infection and is characterized by chronic wasting and emaciation. The visceral granulomas present externally and internally are often composed of a thick capsule of epithelioid cells surrounding necrotic centers containing large numbers of acid-fast bacilli.[25,26,36] Langhans' giant cells and mineralization are rarely encountered in piscine mycobacteriosis.[14,26] Melanocytes are often scattered among the epithelioid cells of the granuloma.[31] A piscine granuloma with pigmented histiocytic cells is shown in **Fig. 1**.

Once mycobacteria become established in an aquarium it may be necessary to destroy all the fish, break down the system, sterilize salvageable material, and start again. The organism can be identified in food, aquarium decorations, plants, and invertebrates in these closed systems, which can explain the high incidence.[19] It is noteworthy that superficial body tissues and internal organs of fish may become contaminated or colonized from a contaminated aqueous environment; however, these isolates are not always associated with clinical disease.[19]

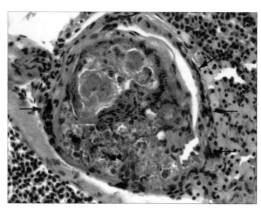

Fig. 1. A piscine granuloma with pigmented histiocytic cells (hematoxylin-eosin, original magnification ×40).

Piscine mycobacteriosis can be a very insidious disease with a long incubation period. Members of the freshwater families Anabantidae (bettas and gouramis), Characidae (tetras and piranhas), and Cyprinidae (danios and barbs) appear to be particularly susceptible.[22,23,38,39] However, some of these fish have a longer survival time in aquariums and this may increase the opportunity for infections.[39] From a large multifacility survey, the common marine species identified with mycobacteria were from the Syngnathid family: leafy seadragon (*Phycodurus eques*), weedy seadragon (*Phyllopteryx taeniolatus*), and various *Hippocampus* species.[29]

Development of vaccines against fish mycobacteriosis have been attempted as fish show a delayed hypersensitivity reaction after immunization with *M salmoniphilum* mixed with Freund's adjuvant.[40] This protection has yet to be achieved.[26]

There are several fish models mimicking a natural mycobacterial infection that enable the study of the pathogen–host interaction.[14,37] The ability of mycobacterium to replicate and survive in macrophages distinguishes pathogenic from nonpathogenic mycobacteria.[41,42] The intracellular trafficking of *M marinum* is analogous to that of *M tuberculosis* in that they both reside in similar phagocytic compartments.[43] It has been shown that phagosomes containing *M marinum* bacterium do not fuse with lysosomes, the result of which is that the organism is able to survive and replicate in macrophages.[43] Several genes are preferentially expressed in *M marinum* when they reside in host granulomas or macrophages. Two are homologs of *M tuberculosis* PE/PE-PGRS genes, a family encoding numerous repetitive glycine-rich proteins of unknown function. Mutation of two PE-PGRS genes produced *M marinum* strains incapable of replication in macrophages and decreased their persistence in gran ulomas.[44] *M marinum* could therefore prove to be a very useful model system for studying intracellular survival and possibly other host–pathogen interactions associated with mycobacterial diseases.[14]

AMPHIBIAN MYCOBACTERIOSIS

Mycobacteriosis in amphibians usually presents as a disease of the integument. It is generally considered secondary to skin wounds. Mycobacteria are present in most aquatic environments and ingestion is also a proven route of infection in tadpoles. Grossly the presenting sign is multiple gray nodules in any or all organs.[45]

Mycobacteria are commonly isolated from a number of captive amphibian species, most often from adult anurans. The species of mycobacteria isolated from amphibians have included *M marinum*, *M chelonei*, *M fortuitum*, *M xenopi*, *M abscessus*, *M avium*, and *M szulgai*.[46,47] Other authors indicate that *M fortuitum*, *M xenopi*, and *M marinum* are the usual organisms isolated from amphibians.[46] Mycobacteriosis is generally a chronic disease that presents with a wide range of clinical signs and gross findings. Chronic granulomatous inflammation is a hallmark of mycobacteriosis, and lesions may appear grossly as solitary or multifocal nodules in the skin, and may present as miliary lesions. Internally, the liver, spleen, intestines, and kidney may be affected. Misdiagnoses of "lymphosarcoma" and "transmissible lymphosarcoma" are often made in cases of amphibian mycobacteriosis. This infection should be a primary differential diagnosis when granulomatous, histiocytic, lymphocytic, caseous, or pyogranulomatous nodules are found in any organ. There is no reported effective treatment of amphibian mycobacteriosis, and the culling of affected animals and thorough disinfection of holding facilities are recommended.[47]

Possibly because they are widely used in laboratories, *Xenopus* sp frogs are described most commonly with mycobacteriosis. A case of cutaneous nodular infection caused by *M gordonae* was seen in a colony of African clawed frogs (*Xenopus tropicalis*). Macroscopic lesions were present only in the skin. Multiple raised cutaneous nodules of various sizes were noted in different body locations. Microscopically, acid-fast bacilli were seen within the cutaneous inflammation of several lesions. In particular, many bacilli were present in the granulomatous inflammation on the skin surface. The lesions were characterized by subcutaneous nodular inflammation comprising predominately macrophages and lymphocytes. Clinical presentation and pathology of *M gordonae* infection in this colony was consistent with the presentation previously observed in human patients. *M gordonae* is usually considered a nonpathogenic commensal found in soil and water and is considered an occasional human pathogen, especially with immunocompromised patients.[48]

During regular health status monitoring, a colony of amphibians, *M gordonae*, was isolated from granulomatous lesions of the toes of the South African clawed frog (*Xenopus laevis*). During a period of 3 years, a total of 21 animals of the colony were affected.[49]

Fig. 2 shows a green frog (*Rana clamitans*) with swelling and necrosis of the toes due to a mycobacterial infection.

A colony of captive African clawed frogs (*Xenopus tropicalis*) became infected with *M szulgai*. Clinical signs, when observed, were lethargy, weight loss, and emaciation.

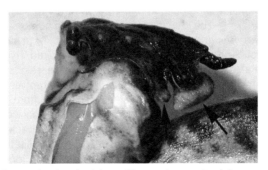

Fig. 2. Green frog (*Rana clamitans*) with swelling and necrosis of the toes due to a mycobacterial infection.

Visceral granulomas were seen at laparoscopy and necropsy. The diagnosis of mycobacteriosis was based on histologic appearance and Ziehl-Neelsen staining of tissues. The identification of *M szulgai* organisms was based on comparison of the 16S rRNA gene sequence with several GenBank databases. There have been no reports of this mycobacterial species as the causative agent of naturally occurring disease in amphibians.[50] Other species of frogs and toads have also been reported to be infected. A colony housing several species of frogs with excessive mortality had hydrocelom and anasarca secondary to glomerulonephritis. The glomerulonephritis was due to chronic infection by mycobacteria.[51]

A captive marine toad, *Bufo marinus*, presented with a spontaneous acute fracture of the left tibia. In spite of amputation and antibacterial therapy, the toad's condition declined and it was euthanized and necropsied. Microscopic evaluation of the fracture site and additional organs found granulomatous inflammation associated with numerous acid-fast positive bacilli. *M marinum* and *M terrae* were isolated from lung and liver.[52]

In a review of amphibian mycobacterial infections diagnosed at the authors' service, the incidence was 1% of total amphibians examined. The frog species included dart frogs (Dendrobatidae), ornate horned frogs (*Ceratophrys ornata*), smoky jungle frogs (*Leptodactylus pentadactylus*), gray tree frogs (*Hyla versicolor*), mossy frogs (*Theloderma corticale*), red-eyed tree frogs (*Agalychnis callidryas*), and golden sedge frogs (*Hyperolius puncticulatus*). Three anurans were infected: Spanish ribbed newt (*Pleurodeles waltl*) and two unspeciated newts. Only one isolate in a red-eyed tree frog (*Agalychnis callidryas*) was further characterized as *M marinum* by PCR.

Experimentally, *M marinum* infection of poikilothermic animals, such as frogs, results in chronic granulomatous diseases that bear many similarities to mycobacterioses in mammals, including tuberculosis. Experimental *M marinum* infection can be used to study basic aspects of *Mycobacterium*–host interactions and granuloma development.[41,42]

REPTILE MYCOBACTERIOSIS

Mycobacterial infections in reptile species are uncommon, occurring only sporadically in captive specimens. The reported incidence of mycobacterial infections has ranged from 0.1% to 1.1% from various collections and studies.[53–56] These infections have been reported in a wide variety of reptiles (snakes, turtles, lizards, and crocodiles), encompassing 24 species. From the literature, the reptilian isolates identified by bacterial growth or PCR have included *M marinum*, *M chelonae*, *M thamnopheos*, *M fortuitum*, *M smegmatis*, *M phlei*, *M haemophilum*, *M intracellulare*, *M kansasii*, *M confluentis*, *M szulgai*, *M hiberniae*, *M neoarum*, *M nonchromogenicum*, *M agri*, *M avium*, and *M ulcerans*.[56,57] The identified isolates from the authors' service include *M chelonae*, *M marinum*, *M kumamotonerse*, *M kansasii*, and *M haemophilum*.[55]

These opportunistic organisms are likely to be acquired by the ingestion of contaminated material (particularly fish or amphibians) or via lesions in the respiratory, integumentary, or urogenital systems. Infections in captive reptiles are suspected to occur because of a repressed immune system, frequently from mismanaged and poorly maintained environmental conditions and poor physical condition (malnutrition). Based on the rare numbers of definitive reports of mycobacteria being isolated from free-ranging populations, this supports that animals debilitated in captivity are particularly susceptible. MOTT (the isolates most commonly identified in reptiles) normally live in soil and aquatic habitats, and most of them are saprophytes. Mycobacterioses in turtles probably originate from contaminated water,[58] and some species such as *M kansasii* have been isolated from water pipe lines and tap water in both the United States and Europe.[17]

The clinical signs in reptiles are nonspecific but can include anorexia or emaciation as well as the identification of firm masses and swellings in the oral cavity or on the body.

The gross appearance of a mycobacterial lesion is of grayish-white nodules in many of the organs as well as in the subcutis. In necropsy reports of mycobacteriosis in reptiles, heterophilic and histiocytic granulomas have been most commonly associated with the lung, liver, kidney, spleen, oral cavity, heart, joints, and subcutaneous locations.[55,59]

On histologic evaluation, the granulomas have a typical appearance of granulomatous inflammation composed of multinucleated giant cells, macrophages, and a variable inflammatory cell population including heterophils, lymphocytes, and plasma cells. The granulomas can range from nodules of viable and degenerate heterophils or nodules with a central core of necrosis surrounded by epithelioid macrophages, multinucleated cells, and a variable mantel of mixed inflammatory cells. It is rare for calcification to occur with reptilian mycobacterial granulomas as has been described in mammalian species. Chronic granulomas are characterized by epithelioid cells, lymphocytes, plasma cells, and eventually multinucleated giant cells surrounding the central lesion. Older granulomas are additionally walled off by fibrous connective tissue.[60]

Reptiles react to many infections by developing granulomatous inflammations that may be classified as heterophilic or histiocytic, depending on the etiology and the host's cellular response.[60] In at least one study,[61] histologic classification of the type of granulomatous inflammation and association specifically to mycobacterial organisms could not be supported. Grouping etiologic agents by either the extracellular or intracellular bacteria with heterophilic or histiocytic granulomas, respectively, did not prove to be consistent.[61] Heterophilic granuloma in a reptile is shown in **Fig. 3**.

The simple isolation of mycobacteria alone does not necessarily indicate disease, as again, they are commonly found in the environment.[62] In one study evaluating the normal oral flora of healthy snakes, *Mycobacterium* was a rare isolate without evidence of clinical disease.[63]

Snakes

In snakes, both oral lesions and pneumonia are common with mycobacterial infections.[12,55,61,64–71] It could be speculated that oral lesions occurred secondary to husbandry issues such as inappropriate caging, handling, or dietary materials,

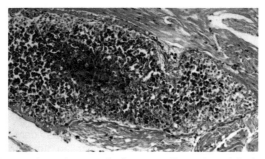

Fig. 3. Heterophilic granuloma in a reptile (hematoxylin-eosin, original magnification ×40).

traumatizing the oral cavity and permitting the mycobacterial infection, which can then, with time, spread specifically to the lungs. This may be due to the oral lesions commonly involving the glottis, which is located cranial in the mouth and with aspiration of inflammatory exudates can result in secondary respiratory infections.[72]

One strain of *M marinum* was isolated from infected snakes and bullfrogs housed in adjacent exhibits over 14 years until it was closed. Utensils and snake hooks were used in both exhibits without cleaning between uses, leading to contamination of the enclosures.[69]

Snakes comprised the majority of reptile mycobacterial cases examined at the authors' service: *Gonyosoma frenatum*, garter snake (*Thamnophis* spp), kingsnake (*Lampropeltis* spp), tentacled (*Erpeton tentaculatum*), Haitian tree boa (*Epicrates gracilis*), emerald tree boa (*Corallus caninus*), horned adder (*Bitis caudalis*), and rattlesnakes (*Crotalus scutulatus* and *C atrox*). All snakes had disseminated disease. *M kansasii* was the isolate from the *Gonyosoma frenatum* and *M chelonae* was present in the Mojave and Western rattlesnakes.[55]

Lizards

Mycobacterial infections in reports from lizards tend to describe disseminated diseases.[55,62,73] It was also noted that some of the infections presented locally with oropharyngeal lesions[55] or lesions of the limbs/joints.[73–75] Breeching the integument (trauma) or the digestive tract seems the most likely route of infection. Some cases were also due to exposure from a contaminated environment or from the diet. A group of Egyptian spiny-tailed lizards (*Uromastyx aegyptius*) were housed in a tank formerly used for fish and not sterilized. Several lizards became debilitated and suffered thermal burns due to a reluctance to move away from heat lamps. Abscesses developed under the areas of the burns and into the joints of their toes and feet. On postmortem examination these lesions were of a granulomatous infection and *M marinum* was isolated.[75] In one case, a bearded dragon with *M marinum* had been fed dead and dying guppies from a tropical tank. The examined guppies also had *M marinum*.[73]

From the authors' service, five lizards (two bearded dragons [*Pogona vitticeps*], a veiled chameleon, [*Chamaeleo calyptratus*], and two common green iguanas [*Iguana iguana*]) were identified with mycobacteriosis. Two of the lizards (bearded dragon and iguana) presented with oropharyngeal lesions. The other three lizards had disseminated disease. *M chelonae* was identified in the veiled chameleon and an iguana. One bearded dragon had *M marinum* and one iguana, *M kumamotonerse*.[55]

Chelonians

In chelonians, mycobacteriosis have been associated with pulmonary and hepatic tubercles, plastronal ulcerations, and granulomatous skin lesions.[76,77] In a Kemp's Ridley sea turtle (*Lepidochelys kempii*),[78] a leatherback sea turtle (*Dermochelys coriacea*),[79] and side-neck turtle (*Phrynops hilari*)[76] the infection was believed to gain entry via skin lesions and spread hematogenously. A Chinese soft-shell turtle (*Pelodiscus sinensis*) developed small white foci on its carapace and within months became anorectic and developed respiratory distress.[17] The lesions supporting mycobacteriosis were of granulomas within the skin of the neck, carapace, and lung.[17] From a survey of farmed marine turtles (*Chelonia mydas*), focal pneumonia due to *Mycobacterium* spp was identified.[80]

An atypical mycobacterial infection, *M ulcerans*, was identified by PCR and nucleotide sequence analysis in an Indian flap-shelled turtle (*Lissemys punctata punctata*) from an aquarium. At necropsy, the turtle had multiple white nodules on the capsular surface and parenchyma of various organs (liver, spleen, intestine, and lung). Histologically, the lesions were typical for a mycobacterial infection with granulomatous inflammation surrounding a central core of necrosis and numerous acid-fast bacilli within intracellular macrophages and the area of central necrosis.[20]

The tortoises recognized in the authors' service with mycobacteriosis were fly river (*Carettochelys insculpta*), Blanding's (*Emydoidea blandingii*), red bellied (*Pseudemys rubriventris*), and Russian tortoise (*Testudo horsfieldii*). Three of the four chelonians had disseminated disease. One presented with a granuloma on the tongue. *M marinum* was isolated from the fly river turtle and *M haemophilum* was isolated from the Russian tortoise.[55]

Crocodilians

M szulgai, an uncommon species of mycobacteria, was isolated from lesions of a granulomatous pneumonia in an adult freshwater crocodile (*Crocodylus johnstoni*). The animal had died unexpectedly and at necropsy a fibrinous exudate in the right pleural cavity and white miliary nodules in the right lung lobe were identified. Histologically, the well demarcated granulomas were typical for the lesion in reptiles, consisting of multinucleated giant cells and epithelioid cells surrounded by fibrous connective tissue. Mycobacterial infection was confirmed by nested PCR targeting the *hsp65* gene and by Fite's method for detection of acid-fast bacilli within formalin-fixed, paraffin-embedded lung tissue.[57]

Probable mycobacterial skin lesions were identified in a survey of skin lesions on farmed Australian crocodiles at a prevalence of 2.5%.[81] The gross lesions were individual, raised, red to gray nodules, on the snout, conjunctiva, jaws, and along the ventral side of the neck and medial thigh. Histologic examination identified a spectrum of lesions from well circumscribed granulomas in the dermis to erosive dermatitis with accumulations of multinucleate giant cells, histiocytes, lymphocytes, and heterophils. Acid-fast organisms in Ziehl-Neelsen–stained sections were scattered throughout the inflammation; however, further identification was not pursued.[81]

Twelve freshwater crocodiles held for study had systemic (lungs, liver, spleen, and kidney) granulomatous infection.[82] The only noted clinical sign was anorexia. In Ziehl-Neelsen–stained sections of the lesion there were numerous acid-fast deposits in the central eosinophilic zones and within giant cells. The diagnosis was made via PCR, but no specific species was reported. These juveniles were likely to have been stressed by repeated handling or winter temperatures.[82] A rare generalized *M avium* infection has been reported in Nile crocodiles (*Crocodylus niloticus*) that had been fed the carcasses of infected pigs.[83] Four rough-eyed caimans (*Caiman sclerops*) had disseminated lesions (lungs, spleen, liver, kidney, pancreas, testis, and epiglottis) due to *M marinum*.[70]

Reptiles have not been used as animal models to study mycobacteria.

RODENT MYCOBACTERIOSIS

Spontaneous mycobacteriosis is very rare in gerbils, mice, hamsters, and guinea pigs and is not associated with a specific mycobacterial species.[46] Case reports of natural disease in rodents included a pet Korean squirrel (*Sciuris vulgaris coreae*), a grizzled giant squirrel (*Ratufa macroura*), and a golden hamster (*Mesocricetus auratus*).[84–86] The Korean squirrel developed a disseminated mycobacterial infection. Grossly, multiple small nodules were noted in the lung, liver, spleen, and skin. Calcification was seen in an enlarged bronchial lymph node. Microscopically, there was a disseminated granulomatous infection. Acid-fast bacilli were detected in macrophages, giant cells, and in some lymphatic vessels. *M avium* subsp *avium* was isolated and identified via

PCR-restriction endonuclease analysis.[84] The pet golden hamster developed spontaneous disseminated mycobacteriosis and presented with enlarged feet and lymph nodes.[85] Granulomatous inflammation with acid-fast bacilli were found in affected tissues microscopically. *M chelonei* was isolated from the foot lesion. In another report, a disseminated infection with *M genavense* was diagnosed in an adult grizzled giant squirrel. Granulomatous inflammation was found in the brain, kidneys, lungs, and maxilla. *M genavense* and a novel species of *Mycobacterium* (proposed name, *Mycobacterium lipsiensis*) were identified.[86]

From submissions of 3078 rodents to the authors' laboratory, only one case of granulomatous pneumonia due to acid-fast positive bacteria was identified in a spiny mouse (*Acomys* sp) from a zoo collection.

Mycobacterial disease has been seen in wild rodents including voles and wood mice.[87] *M microti* is the primary cause of these infections. This organism may spread to other mammals and to humans in some instances.

Although rodents can be used as animal models for mycobacteriosis, mice have proved to be a poor experimental model of mycobacterial infection.[88] However, in the case of *M haemophilum*, mice given prednisone and intravenous injections of the organisms developed ear lesions that were grossly similar to the cutaneous lesions seen in the sporadic human infections.[89]

RABBIT MYCOBACTERIOSIS

Spontaneous mycobacteriosis in rabbits is considered very rare and has not been associated with a specific mycobacterial species.[46]

In one case report an affected rabbit presented sneezing excessively and violently. Endoscopy indicated an excessive amount of crusty, scab-like material in the nasal passages. Tissue was cultured and the organism was identified as one of the *M avium* complex. This particular rabbit had a chronic disease, despite treatment; it was first diagnosed in 2002 and still affected in 2006.[90]

Disseminated mycobacteriosis due to *M avium* was the most common cause of death in a group of adult captive pygmy rabbits. Between June 2002 and September 2004, mycobacteriosis was diagnosed in 28 captive adult pygmy rabbits, representing 29% of the captive population. Compromised cell-mediated immunity appeared to be the best explanation for the high morbidity and mortality associated with mycobacterial infections in these rabbits.[91]

Rabbits have been extensively used as experimental models of mycobacterial infection.[92,93]

FERRET MYCOBACTERIOSIS

Feral ferrets (*Mustela putorius furo*) in New Zealand are considered potential vectors of *M bovis*, being infected after eating contaminated carcasses. Infection causes anorexia, weight loss, and death. Bovine mycobacterial strains lead to a disseminated disease in ferrets, but avian and human strains usually cause slow-growing lesions. Grossly granulomatous lesions may be found radiographically, and are present at necropsy. Antemortem testing has been done experimentally using killed *M tuberculosis* in Freund's complete adjuvant.[94]

Intestinal mycobacteriosis is a rare condition in ferrets. In these cases, the gastrointestinal tract and mesenteric lymph nodes are primarily affected, with mesenteric lymphadenopathy most commonly seen grossly. Histologically, large foamy macrophages with a gray, somewhat granular cytoplasm is noted and acid-fast stains reveal numerous bacilli in the cytoplasm of macrophages.[95,96] Chronic granulomatous

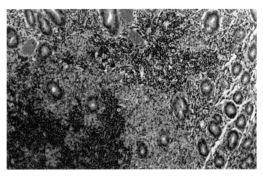

Fig. 4. Granulomatous enteritis in a ferret (hematoxylin-eosin, original magnification ×40).

enteritis in ferrets caused by an acid-fast organism morphologically similar to *M paratuberculosis* has been reported.[97] A similar case has been identified at the authors' laboratory with a granulomatous enteritis (**Fig. 4**) due to an uncharacterized acid fast bacterium (**Fig. 5**).

M genavense infection has been diagnosed in two adult ferrets. Disseminated mycobacteriosis was seen in a castrated 5-year-old ferret including a proliferative lesion of the conjunctiva of the nictitating membrane. A 4-year-old female ferret had conjunctival swelling, serous ocular discharge, and swelling of the subcutis of the nasal bridge. Both ferrets were successfully treated and later died as a result of other disease conditions. The authors concluded that conjunctival involvement may be a feature of disseminated mycobacteriosis in the ferret.[98] From submissions of 4744 ferrets to the authors' laboratory one case of granulomatous conjunctivitis due to acid-fast positive bacteria was identified. Granulomatous otitis externa due to acid-fast bacteria has also been reported.[99]

Mycobacteriosis has been induced in ferrets experimentally.[100] In this study weight loss was most severe with *M bovis* infections. *M bovis* produced more severe gross and histologic lesions than *M avium*, and *M avium* was not consistently recovered from infected animals although *M bovis* was.

SUMMARY

Mycobacteria differ greatly in their ecology, from the obligate pathogen *M tuberculosis*, which is a leading cause of human mortality worldwide, to saprophytic soil

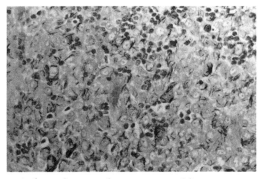

Fig. 5. Acid-fast bacteria from the granulomatous enteritis.

residents such as *M terrae*.[2] Studying the disease in animals may aid in understanding the pathogenesis of mycobacterial infections in humans and identify better therapy and preventative options such as vaccines.

ACKNOWLEDGMENTS

The authors thank Veterinary Information Network for reference support.

REFERENCES

1. Euzéby JP. List of prokaryotic names with standing in nomenclature - genus *Mycobacterium*. Available at: http://www.bacterio.cict.fr/m/mycobacterium.html. Accessed November 15, 2011.
2. Gauthier DT, Rhodes MW. Mycobacteriosis in fishes: a review. Vet J 2009;180(1): 33–47.
3. Rastogi N, Legrand E, Sola C. The mycobacteria: an introduction to nomenclature and pathogenesis. Rev Sci Tech 2001;20:21–54.
4. Tønjum T, Welty DB, Jantzen E, et al. Differentiation of *Mycobacterium ulcerans*, *M. marinum*, and *M. haemophilum*: mapping of their relationships to *M. tuberculosis* by fatty acid profile analysis, DNA-DNA hybridization, and 16S rRNA gene sequence analysis. J Clin Microbiol 1998;36(4):918–25.
5. Bercovier H, Vincent V. Mycobacterial infections in domestic and wild animals due to *Mycobacterium marinum*, *M. fortuitum*, *M. chelonae*, *M. porcinum*, *M. farcinogenes*, *M. smegmatis*, *M. scrofulaceum*, *M. xenopi*, *M. kansasii*, *M. simiae* and *M. genavense*. Rev Sci Tech 2001;20(1):265–90.
6. Runyon EH. Anonymous mycobacteria in pulmonary disease. Med Clin North Am 1959;43(1):273–90.
7. Pourahmad F, Thompson KD, Adams A, et al. Detection and identification of aquatic mycobacteria in formalin-fixed, paraffin-embedded fish tissues. J Fish Dis 2009;32(5): 409–19.
8. Jacobs JM, Stine CB, Baya AM, et al. A review of mycobacteriosis in marine fish. J Fish Dis 2009;32(2):119–30.
9. Kaattari IM, Rhodes MW, Kaattari SL, et al. The evolving story of *Mycobacterium tuberculosis* clade members detected in fish. J Fish Dis 2006;29(9):509–20.
10. Pourahmad F, Thompson KD, Taggart JB, et al. Evaluation of the INNO-LiPA mycobacteria v2 assay for identification of aquatic mycobacteria. J Fish Dis 2008;31: 931–40.
11. BSAVA's Scientific Committee. Tuberculosis. J Small Anim Pract 1999;40(3):145–7.
12. Hernandez-Divers SJ, Shearer D. Pulmonary mycobacteriosis caused by *Mycobacterium haemophilum* and *M. marinum* in a royal python. J Am Vet Med Assoc 2002;220(11):1661–3.
13. Huminer D, Pitlik SD, Block C, et al. Aquarium-borne *Mycobacterium marinum* skin infection. Report of a case and review of the literature. Arch Dermatol 1986;122(6): 698–703.
14. Decostere A, Hermans K, Haesebrouck F. Piscine mycobacteriosis: a literature review covering the agent and the disease it causes in fish and humans. Vet Microbiol 2004;99(3–4):159–66.
15. Saubolle MA, Kiehn TE, White MH, et al. *Mycobacterium haemophilum*: microbiology and expanding clinical and geographic spectra of disease in humans. Clin Microbiol Rev 1996;9:435–47.
16. Shojaei H, Heidarieh P, Hashemi A, et al. Species identification of neglected nontuberculous mycobacteria in a developing country. Jpn J Infect Dis 2011;64:265–71.

17. Oros J, Acosta B, Gaskin JM, et al. *Mycobacterium kansasii* infection in a Chinese soft shell turtle (*Pelodiscus sinensis*). Vet Rec 2003;152(15):474–6.
18. Winthrop KL. Pulmonary disease due to nontuberculous mycobacteria: an epidemiologist's view. Future Microbiol 2010;5(3):343–5.
19. Beran V, Matlova L, Dvorska L, et al. Distribution of mycobacteria in clinically healthy ornamental fish and their aquarium environment. J Fish Dis 2006;29(7):383–93.
20. van der Werf TS, Stienstra Y, Johnson RC, et al. *Mycobacterium ulcerans* disease. Bull World Health Organ 2005;83(10):785–91.
21. Sakaguchi K, Iima H, Hirayama K, et al. *Mycobacterium ulcerans* infection in an Indian flap-shelled turtle (*Lissemys punctata punctata*). J Vet Med Sci 2011;73(9):1217–20.
22. Conroy D. A report on the problems of bacterial fish diseases in the Argentine Republic. Bull Off Int Epizoot 1966;65:755–68.
23. Nigrelli RF, Vogel H. Spontaneous tuberculosis in fishes and in other cold-blooded vertebrates with special reference to *Mycobacterium fortuitum* Cruz from fish and human lesions. Zoologica 1963;48:131–44.
24. Gomez S. Prevalence of microscopic tubercular lesions in freshwater ornamental fish exhibiting clinical signs of non-specific chronic disease. Dis Aquat Organ 2008;80(2):167–71.
25. Smith SA. Mycobacterial infections in pet fish. Semin Avian Exotic Pet Med 1997;6(1):40–5.
26. Chinabut S, Mycobacteriosis and nocardiosis. In: Woo PTK, Bruno DW, editors. Fish diseases and disorders, vol. 3. New York: CABI; 1999. p. 319–40.
27. Francis-Floyd R, Yanong R. Mycobacteriosis in fish. Available at: http://edis.ifas.ufl.edu/VM055. Accessed May 23, 2011.
28. Macri D, Lo Verde V, Mancuso I, et al. Mycobacteriosis in ornamental fish. Case reports in Sicily and medical-legal considerations. Vet Res Commun 2008;32(Suppl 1):S215–7.
29. Kilgore KH, Zollinger TJ, Yanong RPE. Mycobacteriosis in zoos and public aquaria: updated summary and report of a survey concerning incidence, surveillance,and treatment. In: Proceedings of the International Association for Aquatic Animal Medicine. Orlando (FL); 2007. p. 188–9.
30. Frerichs GN. Bacterial diseases of marine fish. Vet Rec 1989;125(12):315–8.
31. Noga EJ, Wright JF, Pasarell L. Some unusual features of mycobacteriosis in the cichlid fish *Oreochromis mossambicus*. J Comp Pathol 1990;102(3):335–44.
32. Parisot TJ, Wood JN. Fish mycobacteriosis (tuberculosis). Fish disease leaflet (No. 7). Washington, DC: Department of the Interior, U.S. Fish and Wildlife Service; 1970.
33. Anderson P, Petty BD. Mixed metazoan and bacterial infection of the gas bladder of the lined seahorse, *Hippocampus erectus*: a case report. In: Proceedings of the International Association for Aquatic Animal Medicine. Orlando (FL); 2007. p. 36–7.
34. Harriff MJ, Bermudez LE, Kent ML. Experimental exposure of zebrafish 'Danio rerio Hamilton' to *Mycobacterium marinum* and *Mycobacterium peregrinum* reveals the gastrointestinal tract as the primary route of infection: a potential model for environmental mycobacterial infection. J Fish Dis 2007;29:1–13.
35. Frerichs GN. Mycobacteriosis: nocardiosis. In: Inglis V, Roberts RJ, Bromage NR, editors. Bacterial diseases of fish. London: Blackwell; 1993. p. 219–35.
36. Grady AW, Wolff A, Besch-Williford C. Diagnostic exercise: visceral granulomas in a fish. Lab Anim Sci 1992;42(3):316–7.
37. Talaat AM, Reimschuessel R, Wasserman SS, et al. Goldfish, *Carassius auratus*, a novel animal model for the study of *Mycobacterium marinum* pathogenesis. Infect Immun 1998;66:2938–42.

38. Astrofsky KM, Schrenzel MD, Bullis RA, et al. Diagnosis and management of atypical *Mycobacterium* spp. infections in established laboratory zebrafish (*Brachydanio rerio*) facilities. Comp Med 2000;50(6):666–72.

39. Speare DJ. Liver diseases of tropical fish. Semin Avian Exotic Pet Med 2000;9(3): 174–8.

40. Bartos JM, Sommer CV. In vivo cell mediated immune response to *M. tuberculosis* and *M. salmoniphilum* in rainbow trout. Dev Comp Immun 1981;5:75–83.

41. Ramakrishnan L, Valdivia RH, McKerrow JH, et al. *Mycobacterium marinum* causes both long-term subclinical infection and acute disease in the leopard frog (*Rana pipiens*). Infect Immun 1997;65:767–73.

42. Cosma CJ, Swaim LE, Volkman H, et al. Zebrafish and frog models of *Mycobacterium marinum* infection. Curr Protoc Microbiol 2006;10(Unit 10B):2.

43. Barker LP, Brooks DM, Small PLC. The identification of *Mycobacterium marinum* genes differentially expressed in macrophage phagosomes using promoter fusions to green fluorescent protein. Mol Microbiol 1998;29:1167–77.

44. Ramakrishnan L, Federspiel NA, Falkow S. Granuloma-specific expression of *Mycobacterium* virulence proteins from the glycine-rich PE-PGRS family. Science 2000; 288:1436–9.

45. Taylor SK, Green DE, Wright KM, et al. Bacterial diseases. In: Wright DM, Whitaker BR, editors. Amphibian medicine and captive husbandry. Malabar (FL): Krieger; 2001. p. 167–9.

46. Hoop RK. Mycobacterial infections. Semin Avian Exotic Pet Med 1997;6:3–8.

47. Densmore CL, Green E. Diseases of amphibians. ILAR J 2007;48:235–54.

48. Sanchez-Morgado JM, Gallagher A, Johnson LK. *Mycobacterium gordonae* infection in a colony of African clawed frogs (*Xenopus tropicalis*). Lab Anim 2009;43:300–3.

49. Kirsch P, Nusser P, Hotzel H, et al. *Mycobacterium gordonae* as potential cause of granulomatous lesions of the toe tips in the South African clawed frog (*Xenopus laevis*). Berl Munch Tierarztl Wochenschr 2008;121:270–7.

50. Chai N, Deforges L, Sougakoff W, et al. *Mycobacterium szulgai* infection in a captive population of African clawed frogs (*Xenopus tropicalis*). J Zoo Wildl Med 2006;37: 55–8.

51. Vannevel JY. Glomerulonephritis and anasarca in a colony of frogs. Vet Clin Exot Anim 2006;9:609–16.

52. Fitzgerald SD, de Maar TWJ, Thomas JS, et al. Pathologic limb fracture attributed to mycobacterial infection in a marine toad, *Bufo marinus*, with systemic mycobacteriosis and chromomycosis. J Herpetol Med Surg 2004;14(3):19–23.

53. Cowan DF. Diseases of captive reptiles. J Am Vet Med Assoc 1968;153:848–59.

54. Jacobson ER. Bacterial disease of reptiles. In: Jacobson ER, editor. Infectious diseases and pathology of reptiles: color atlas and text. Boca Raton (FL): CRC Press; 2007. p. 468–9.

55. Reavill D, Schmidt R, Bradway D. Mycobacterial infections in reptiles. In: Proceedings of the Association of Reptilian and Amphibian Veterinarians. South Padre Island (TX); 2010. p. 16–7.

56. Hoop RK. Public health implications of exotic pet mycobacteriosis. Semin Avian Exotic Pet Med 1997;6(1):3–8.

57. Roh YS, Park H, Cho A, et al. Granulomatous pneumonia in a captive freshwater crocodile (*Crocodylus johnstoni*) caused by *Mycobacterium szulgai*. J Zoo Wildl Med. 2010;41(3):550–4.

58. Brownstein DG. Mycobacteriosis. In: Hoff GL, Frye FL, Jacobson ER, editors. Diseases of amphibians and reptiles. New York: Plenum Press; 1984. p. 1–23.

59. Frye FL. Infectious diseases, fungal, actinomycete, bacterial, rickettsial and viral diseases. In: Frye FL, editor. Biomedical and surgical aspects of captive reptile husbandry. 2nd edition. Malabar (FL): Krieger; 1991. p. 101–60.
60. Montali RJ. Comparative pathology of inflammation in the higher vertebrates (reptiles, birds and mammals). J Comp Pathol 1988;99:1–26.
61. Soldati G, Lu ZH, Vaughan L, et al. Detection of mycobacteria and chlamydiae in granulomatous inflammation of reptiles: a retrospective study. Vet Pathol 2004;41(4): 388–97.
62. Friend SC, Russell EG. Mycobacterium intracellulare infection in a water monitor. J Wildl Dis 1979;15(2):229–33.
63. Draper CS, Walker RD, Lawler HE. Patterns of oral bacterial infection in captive snakes. J Am Vet Med Assoc 1981;179(11):1223–6.
64. Kiel JL. Reptilian tuberculosis in a boa constrictor. J Zoo Anim Med 1977;8:9–11.
65. Olson GA, Woodward JC. Miliary tuberculosis in a reticulated python. J Am Vet Med Assoc 1974;164:733–5.
66. Jacobson ER. Diseases of the respiratory system in reptiles. Vet Med Small Anim Clin 1978;73(9):1169–75.
67. Quesenberry KE, Jacobson ER, Allen JL, et al. Ulcerative stomatitis and subcutaneous granulomas caused by *Mycobacterium chelonei* in a boa constrictor. J Am Vet Med Assoc 1986;189(9):1131–2.
68. Olson GI, Hodgin C, Peckman R. Infectious stomatitis associated with *Mycobacterium* sp, in a boa constrictor. Comp Anim Pract 1987;8:47–9.
69. Maslow JN, Wallace R, Michaels M, et al. Outbreak of *Mycobacterium marinum* infection among captive snakes and bullfrogs. Zoo Biol 2002;21:233–41.
70. Griffith AS. Tuberculosis in captive wild animals. J Hyg (Lond) 1928;28(2):198–218.
71. Aronson JD. Spontaneous tuberculosis in snakes. J Infect Dis 1929;44:215–23.
72. Mehler SJ, Bennett RA. Oral, dental, and beak disorders of reptiles. Vet Clin North Am Exot Anim Pract 2003;6(3):477–503.
73. Girling SJ, Fraser MA. Systemic mycobacteriosis in an inland bearded dragon (*Pogona vitticeps*). Vet Rec 2007;160(15):526–8.
74. Kramer MH. Granulomatous osteomyelitis associated with atypical mycobacteriosis in a bearded dragon (*Pogona vitticeps*), Vet Clin North Am Exot Anim Pract 2006;9: 563–8.
75. Morales P, Dunker F. Fish tuberculosis, *Mycobacterium marinum*, in a group of Egyptian spiny-tailed lizards, *Uromastyx aegyptius*. J Herpetol Med Surg 2001;11(3): 27–30.
76. Rhodin AGJ, Anver MR. Mycobacteriosis in turtles: cutaneous and hepatosplenic involvement in a *Phrynops hilari*. J Wildl Diseas 1977;13:180–3.
77. Keymer IF. Diseases of chelonians: (2) necropsy survey of terrapins and turtles. Vet Rec 1978;103(26–27):577–82.
78. Greer LL, Strandberg JD, Whitaker BR. *Mycobacterium chelonae* osteoarthritis in a Kemp's ridley sea turtle, *Lepidochelys kempii*. J Wildl Dis 2003;39(3):736–41.
79. Ogden NA, Rhodin AGJ, Conlogue GJ, et al. Pathobiology of septic arthritis and contiguous osteomyelitis in a leatherback turtle (*Dermochelys coriacea*). J Wildl Dis 1981;17:277–87.
80. Glazebrook JS, Campbell RSF. A survey of the diseases of marine turtles in northern Australia. I. Farmed turtles. Dis Aquat Org 1990;9:83–95.
81. Buenviaje GN, Ladds PW, Martin Y. Pathology of skin diseases in crocodiles. Aust Vet J 1998;76(5):357–63.
82. Ariel E, Ladds PW, Roberts BL. Mycobacteriosis in young freshwater crocodiles (*Crocodylus johnstoni*). Aust Vet J 1997;75(11):831–3.

83. Huchzermeyer FW. Public health risks of ostrich and crocodile meat. Rev Sci Tech 1997;16(2):599–604.
84. Moreno B, Aduriz G, Garrido JM, et al. Disseminated *Mycobacterium avium* subsp. *avium* infection in a pet Korean squirrel (*Sciuris vulgaris coreae*). Vet Pathol 2007;44: 123–5.
85. Karse E. Disseminated mycobacteriosis in the golden hamster. J Vet Med B 1987; 34:391–4.
86. Theuss T, Aupperle H, Eulenberger K, et al. Disseminated infection with *Mycobacterium genavense* in a grizzled giant squirrel (*Ratufa macroura*) associated with the isolation of an unknown *Mycobacterium*. J Comp Pathol 2010;143:195–8.
87. Xavier Emmanuel F, Seagar AL, Doig C, et al. Human and animal infections with *Mycobacterium microti*, Scotland. Emerg Infect Dis 2007;13(12):1924–7.
88. Young D. Animal models of tuberculosis. Eur J Immunol 2009;39:2011–4.
89. Abbott MR, Smith DD. The pathogenic effects of *Mycobacterium haemophilum* in immunosuppressed albino mice. J Med Microbiol 1980;13:535–40.
90. Kelleher SA. Rabbit respiratory diseases. In: Proceedings of the 80th Western Veterinary Conference. Las Vegas (NV), April 15, 2008; v471.
91. Harrenstien LA, Finnegan MV, Woodford NL, et al. *Mycobacterium avium* in pygmy rabbits (*Brachylagus idahoensis*): 28 cases. J Zoo Wildl Med 2006;37:498–512.
92. Adan CBD, Sato EH, Sousa LB, et al. An experimental model of mycobacterial infection under corneal flaps. Braz J Med Biol Res 2004;37:1015–21.
93. Liang Q-F, Wang Z-G, Deng S-J, et al. Experimental study of non-tuberculous mycobacterial keratitis in rabbits. Zhonghua Yan Ke Za Zhi 2007;43:613–7.
94. Lewington JH. Ferret husbandry, medicine and surgery. Philadelphia: Elsevier; 2000. p. 117–8.
95. Anonymous. Pathology of ferret diseases. Available at: www.ferrethealth.msu.edu/Diseases/Notes.pdf. Accessed November 15, 2011.
96. Williams BH. Pathology of the domestic ferret (*Mustela putorius furo*). Available at: www.docstoc.com/docs/50542310/Pathology-of-the-Domestic-Ferret-(-Mustela-putorius-furo. Accessed November 15, 2011.
97. Bryant JL, Hanner TL, Hurley SL, et al. A chronic granulomatons intestinal disease in ferrets caused by an acid-fast organism morphologically similar to *Myobacterium paratuberculosis*. Lab Anim Sci 1988;38:498–9.
98. Lucas A, Furber H, James G, et al. *Mycobacterium genavense* infection in two aged ferrets with conjunctival lesions. Austral Vet J 2000;78:685–9.
99. Garner MM. Focus on diseases of ferrets. In: Proceedings of the International Conference on Exotics. Florida; 2000. p. 80.
100. Cross ML, Labes RE, Mackintosh CG. Oral infection of ferrets with virulent *Mycobacterium bovis* or *Mycobacterium avium*: susceptibility, pathogenesis and immune response. J Comp Pathol 2000;123:15–21.

Pathology of Mycobacteriosis in Birds

H.L. Shivaprasad, BVSc, MS, PhD, DACPV[a],*, Chiara Palmieri, DVM, PhD, DECVP[b]

KEYWORDS

- *Mycobacterium* • Mycobacteriosis • Pathogenesis
- Tuberculosis • Pathology • Cytology • Acid-fast • Amyloid
- Birds • Avian

Mycobacteriosis is one of the most common diseases of various species of birds including domestic poultry, pet and exotic birds such as psittacines and canaries, and free-living and captive wild birds.[1–11] The disease in birds is generally caused by *Mycobacterium avium* subsp *avium,* [6] but more than 10 other species of mycobacteria have been known to infect birds.[12–24] These include *M genavense, M tuberculosis, M bovis, M gordonae, M nonchromogenicum, M fortuitum* subsp *fortuitum, M avium* subsp *hominissuis, M peregrinum, M intermedium, M celatum, M intracellulare, M avium* subsp *paratuberculosis, M africanum,* and *M simiae.*

The oral route of infection appears to be the primary mode of transmission of mycobacteriosis in birds based on the lesions most commonly found in the intestine and liver. In some cases, the extensive involvement of the respiratory system especially lungs suggests an airborne mode of transmission.[4,8,21,25,26] Following oral ingestion, *M avium* initially infects the intestine and, due to lack of lymph nodes in birds, readily spreads to liver, spleen, bone marrow, lungs, air sacs, gonads, and other organs.[7] As the disease progresses, it causes noncaseated, nonmineralized nodules in different organs of most birds. Birds do not form classic tubercles as seen in mammals due to mycobacteriosis. In some cases, masses in the skin and conjunctiva can also be observed. On necropsy, liver and spleen may be enlarged and the proximal intestine may appear tubular, thickened, and tan colored.[27] Microscopically, in most organs the lesions consist of nodules made up of foamy macrophages containing large numbers of acid-fast bacilli (AFB).[3]

The authors have nothing to disclose.
[a] Avian Pathology, California Animal Health and Food Safety Laboratory System–Tulare Branch, University of California, Davis, 18830 Road 112, Tulare, CA 93274, USA
[b] Faculty of Veterinary Medicine, Veterinary Pathology Division, University of Teramo, Piazza Aldo Moro, 45, Teramo, 64100, Italy
* Corresponding author.
E-mail address: hlshivaprasad@ucdavis.edu

PATHOGENESIS OF THE INFECTIOUS PROCESS

The chronic presentation of avian mycobacteriosis results from the prolonged immunologic battle between host, mainly through a cell-mediated immune response, and the pathogen.[10] The key event of this immune failure is the ability of mycobacteria to downregulate killing mechanisms of the macrophages, once phagocytosed, and prevent the normal fusion of the phagosome with lysosomes,[10] even if the precise mechanism of *Mycobacterium* spp survival within avian macrophages is yet unknown.[28] Besides inhibition of phagosome-lysosome fusion, disruption of the phagosome, interference with cytokine synthesis and functions, and inactivation of lysosomal enzymes have been suggested.[29] The pathogenicity of *M avium* has been attributed in part to its unique cell wall, composed of a complex array of hydrocarbon chains containing the arabinogalactan-peptidoglycan mycolic acid core found in all mycobacteria, surrounded by a second layer made up in part of specific glycopeptidolipids (GPLs) found only in *M avium*[30] and responsible for the delayed phagosome-lysosome fusion, similarly to the surface-located mannosylated lipoarabinomannan of *M tuberculosis*.[31] Another important feature of mycobacterial infection is the development of delayed type hypersensitivity (DTH) after 2 days of infection.[32] This response is mediated by lymphocytes that stimulate chemotaxis and activation of macrophages, increases in intensity as the disease progresses, and is inversely related with the severity of the disease.[10] Depending on the host immune response and severity of bacterial replication, 3 stages can be identified in the evolution of the disease in chicken.[32] At 7 days post infection (p.i.), no microscopic lesions are found, only the development of DTH reactions (latency period). Later, during the lesion development stage (8 to 17 p.i.), mycobacteria replicate, small tubercles occur and serum antibody titers develop. Finally, the cachexia period is characterized by massive formation of tubercles with large number of bacteria and deposition of amyloid, lymphoid atrophy and disappearance of DTH.[10] During this period, the classic gross and histopathologic lesions of mycobacteriosis in chicken become evident.

GROSS PATHOLOGY

Gross pathology due to mycobacteriosis in birds can be variable depending on the species of bird affected, stage of the disease (lag phase), age of the bird, concurrent infections, host's immune and nutritional status, and genetics but not necessarily due to the species of mycobacteria.

One of the most commonly observed feature due to mycobacteriosis in birds is poor body condition, with birds appearing thin or emaciated and evident atrophy of pectoral muscles with a prominent keel in many species of birds, especially in backyard domestic poultry (**Fig. 1**).[1,10] Often there is loss of fat reserves in the subcutis, abdominal cavity, and coronary groove of the heart, and occasionally serous atrophy of fat can be observed.[33] Pale carcasses suggesting anemia due to mycobacteriosis have been observed occasionally in birds.[6]

External lesions compared to the internal lesions due to mycobacteriosis are not common in birds but have been observed. These include subcutaneous swellings that can appear as tumors.[34–38] Most of such lesions have been attributed to *M tuberculosis* in parrots,[20,34] but other species such as *M genavense*,[36] *M avium* subsp *avium*,[33] and *M avium* subsp *paratuberculosis*[19] can cause similar lesions not only in psittacine but also in other species of birds including quail, falcons, ostriches, and wild birds. Most common skin lesions are small cutaneous nodules ranging in size from a few millimeters to 1 cm on the head and face and occasionally in the mandible and neck of psittacines.[39] Some masses as large as 4 cm horny growth have also

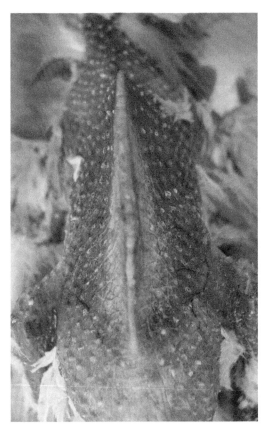

Fig. 1. Ring-necked dove (*Streptopelia risoria*). Severe atrophy of pectoral muscles with prominent keel. (*Courtesy of* Dr Miguel D. Saggese.)

been described in psittacines.[37] In one instance, a subcutaneous discrete mass measuring 20 × 7 cm associated with AFB was removed from the neck region of an apparently healthy 2-year-old female ostrich.[40] Similarly, subcutaneous nodules due to mycobacteriosis can also be observed on the legs and wings and occasionally on the abdomen and dorsum of the body in various species of birds.[37,41] In another study of Gyr hybrid falcons, yellowish discolored firm cutaneous lesions associated with AFB were found in the thigh and lateral thoracic and abdominal regions in 18 falcons.[41] The subcutaneous nodules usually have a smooth surface but can ulcerate if traumatized. Sometimes these nodules could also be a manifestation of joint or bone infection due to mycobacteriosis.[9]

Other external lesions that have been reported include protrusion of one or both eyes due to retrobulbar mycobacteriosis, nodules in the eye lids including the external canthus, bulbar and palpebral conjunctivae, and nictitating membrane.[34,38,42,43] One unusual manifestation of mycobacteriosis in the eye was the presence of a large mass about the size of a hen's egg (approximately 8 × 5 cm) on the inner conjunctival surface of the lower eye lid in a 2-year-old ostrich that was suffering from ocular and nasal discharge.[44] Other ocular lesions such as keratitis has been described in an adult Maximillian's parrot.[45] A solid red mass protruding from the left ear composed

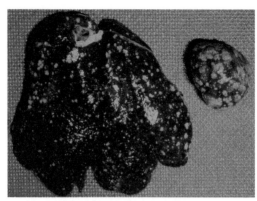

Fig. 2. Chicken (*Gallus gallus*). Moderate hepatomegaly and severe splenomegaly with multifocal to coalescing white-to-yellow nodules.

of granulomas containing AFB has been reported in a blue-headed parrot.[45] Swelling of left infraorbital sinus containing abundant yellow caseous exudate due to mycobacteriosis has been observed in a female kakariki parakeet (*Cyanoramphus* spp). An unusual and rare outbreak of mycobacteriosis due to *M avium* in 48-week-old commercial layer chickens with manifestation of swelling of the infraorbital sinuses has been reported.[46]

Mycobacteriosis in commercial chickens is extremely rare.[6] Pathologic fractures of long bones due to osteomyelitis caused by mycobacteria have been reported in various species of psittacines and wild birds.[1,47] Other nonspecific lesions such as dull or loss of feathers, scaly skin, and pale combs associated with mycobacteriosis have been also described in various species of birds.[48,49]

Internal organs most commonly affected by mycobacteriosis in birds are the liver, spleen, intestines, lungs, air sacs, and thoracic and abdominal cavities.[1,6,10] However, it is not uncommon to find lesions limited to one or a few organs due to mycobacteriosis in birds. The morphology of gross lesions due to mycobacteriosis varies between species of birds. In birds such as chickens, turkeys, pheasants, quail (Galliformes), pigeons (Columbiformes), ratites (Struthioniformes, Rheiformes), raptors (Falconiformes, Accipitrifomes), and other wild birds, the lesions can be obvious. They can manifest as pale yellow white to tan nodules of various sizes in organs such as liver, spleen (**Fig. 2**), intestine (**Fig. 3**), bone marrow, lungs (**Fig. 4**), air sacs, and mesentery.[1,10,50–53] These nodules can range from a few millimeters to 1 to 2 cm or more in diameter present not only on the surface of an organ but also in the parenchyma. Occasionally 90% of the spleen can be involved with such granulomas (**Fig. 5**). Larger nodules are caseous but seldom mineralize.[1,3,54] Other organs such as the upper digestive tract, gonads, heart, skin, and skeletal muscles can be affected but this is considered rare.[55,56] *M avium* was isolated from 2 small pale yellow nodules in the brain of a 21-month-old chicken that had paralysis and other symptoms.[57]

In psittacines and passerines such as canaries, finches, and song birds, the most commonly involved organs are liver, spleen, and intestine.[7,58,59] However, it should be emphasized that gross lesions are not always discernible or obvious in psittacines and in canaries and finches and that unless histopathology, culture, and PCR are performed, the diagnosis of mycobacteriosis can be missed. Gross lesions in the liver can range from mild to moderate diffuse enlargement, which can be either diffusely pale-white or occasionally mottled (**Fig. 6**) with pale-white to tan-brown foci.[60,61]

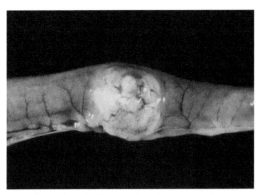

Fig. 3. Peafowl (*Pavo* sp), intestine. Solitary pale-yellow granuloma.

Occasionally, the liver can be enlarged with multiple tan-yellow firm nodules ranging in size from 3 to 5 mm in diameter (**Fig. 7**). In one psittacine, a creamino lineolated parakeet (*Bolborhynchus* sp) the liver was so large that it weighted 20% of the bird's body weight. The spleen is also commonly involved, and it can be mild to severely enlarged and pale or enlarged and mottled white (**Fig. 8**).[62] Gross lesions in the intestine can be mild to severe distentions of the proximal intestine, especially the duodenum and proximal jejunum. The serosa can be pale and the wall severely thickened ("rope-like"). The mucosa can have prominent villi with numerous miliary foci giving it a "shaggy" appearance (**Fig. 9**).[6] Occasionally, the distal intestine can be thin-walled and contain a few pale small miliary nodules.[63] Pale tan or yellow nodules can also be found attached to the peritoneal lining or the mesentery.[53,54] Similar nodules can also be found in the lungs, pleura, thoracic inlet, heart, and air sacs.[42] Some of these nodules appear like tumors such as in a 20-year-old female double yellow-headed Amazon parrot (*Amazona oratrix*) that had a pale-tan large irregular mass measuring 3 × 3 × 3 cm at the base of the heart. Occasionally, the aorta at the base of the heart can be involved and it can appear as a yellow wall.[64,65] An adult cockatiel died due to cardiac tamponade after 2 days' duration of acute dyspnea and had aortal arteritis associated with AFB and atherosclerosis.

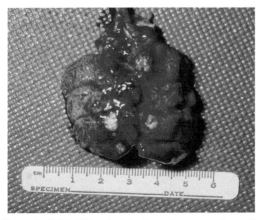

Fig. 4. Chicken (*Gallus gallus*). Multifocal white-to-yellow granulomas in the lung.

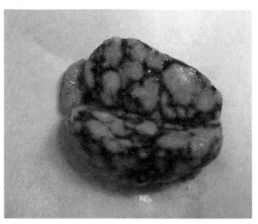

Fig. 5. Ring-necked dove (*Streptopelia risoria*). Cut section of the spleen showing multifocal to coalescing white-to-tan nodules effacing almost completely the splenic parenchyma.

Another condition often associated with mycobacteriosis in certain species of birds such as Anseriformes is amyloidosis.[51] Amyloid is an acute phase protein that accumulates as homogeneous eosinophilic material extracellularly in various organs but most commonly in the liver, spleen, intestine, and adrenal gland. The birds affected with amyloidosis will have mild to severe diffuse enlargement of the liver that can be firm pale or yellow, with a waxy appearance and granulomas of mycobacteriosis scattered here and there. Spleen affected with amyloid can also be diffusely enlarged and pale, with some as much as 5 times the normal size, and contains scattered granulomas.[10] Based on these observations, it has been speculated that amyloidosis is secondary to chronic mycobacteriosis. However, Anseriformes such as ducks have a genetic predisposition to develop amyloidosis.[1,66] Therefore, even though ducks with mycobacteriosis often have amyloid, it is more likely that this is a coincidence. It is possible that mycobacteriosis may enhance amyloid deposition in the liver, spleen, and other organs in ducks. Amyloidosis

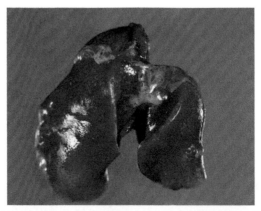

Fig. 6. Blue-headed Pionus parrot (*Pionus menstruus*). Enlarged and mottled white liver. This is the most common manifestation of mycobacteriosis in psittacines.

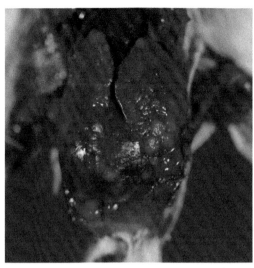

Fig. 7. Grey-cheeked parakeet (*Brotogeris pyrrhoptera*). Multifocal to coalescing yellow nodules within the liver parenchyma.

is a common occurrence in commercial ducks, and it is commonly referred to as "water belly" due to the accumulation of serous fluid in the abdominal cavity. This condition most commonly occurs in adults without any underlying infectious disease, suggesting that it is a metabolic condition likely influenced by genetics. This is supported by the occurrence of amyloidosis in Pekin ducks as young as 4 weeks and not associated with any underlying infectious or noninfectious diseases. Mycobacteriosis has not been reported in commercial Pekin ducks that had amyloidosis. Also, amyloidosis is relatively common in canaries and finches, but there have been no reports of mycobacteriosis occurring in these species of birds in conjunction with amyloidosis (H. L. Shivaprasad, unpublished data, 2011).

Other lesions that have been described due to mycobacteriosis include pale-yellow plaques or nodules in the tongue, oral cavity, larynx, trachea, abdominal air sacs,

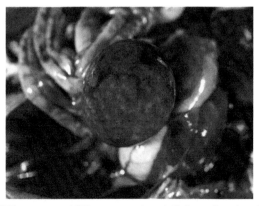

Fig. 8. Blue-headed Pionus parrot (*Pionus menstruus*). Enlarged and mottled white spleen.

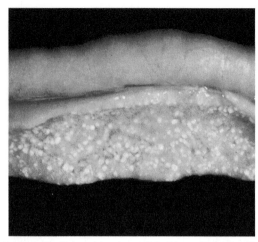

Fig. 9. Moustached parakeet (*Psittacula alexandri*). Disseminated military nodules on the mucosa of the small intestine.

kidneys, pancreas, gizzard, and gonads.[1,12,34,67,68] It should be emphasized that gross lesions of mycobacteriosis in birds are not characteristic, and cytology and histopathology, with the aid of acid-fast stain, can provide rapid and accurate postmortem presumptive diagnosis of mycobacteriosis. However, the exact characterization of the microorganism involved should be pursued by microbiological or, more commonly now, molecular methods.

CYTOLOGY

Impression smears made of a suspected granuloma of mycobacteriosis of the skin, conjunctiva, liver, spleen, intestine, or other organs and stained with Ziehl-Nielsen can reveal large number of AFB in the cytoplasm of macrophages or multinucleated giant cells (**Fig. 10**).[6,7]

HISTOPATHOLOGY

Histopathology combined with acid-fast staining is very helpful for a presumptive diagnosis of mycobacteriosis in birds as the lesions contain numerous AFB.[1]

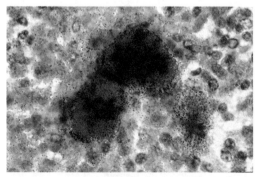

Fig. 10. Cockatiel (*Nymphicus hollandicus*). Impression smear taken from the conjunctiva with macrophages and giant cells containing acid-fast bacteria (Ziehl-Nielsen stain).

However, AFB are nonpathognomonic of the genus *Mycobacterium* and do not confirm the identity of the species involved in the case. We emphasize the need for a definitive molecular characterization of the species of *Mycobacterium*.

Histopathology will reveal more lesions in organs that are not discernible grossly in most organs (disseminated mycobacteriosis). Occasionally, it is not too unusual to see lesions of mycobacteriosis in only one organ such as the skin (localized mycobacteriosis).[1,10] Histologic lesions have been described in almost all organs but most frequently in the intestine, liver, spleen, lung, peritoneum, heart, bone and bone marrow, and skin.[1,10,50,51,69] An interesting lesion, ganglioneuritis of the intestine associated with AFB, has been described in a spectacled Amazon parrot (*Amazona albifrons*).[70] Other organs relatively less commonly affected include eye with conjunctiva, adrenal, kidney, air sac, tongue, skeletal muscle, gonads, thymus, brain, larynx, trachea, pancreas, synovium, sinuses, parathyroid gland, thyroid, and perineurium.[10,50,54,69]

Three types of histologic lesions can be observed depending on the species of birds affected but irrespective of the *Mycobacterium* sp infection.[6] Corresponding to gross lesions seen in certain species of birds such as gallinaceous birds including chickens, turkeys and quail, and pigeons, ratites, raptors, and wild birds including ducks, the lesions are typically granulomas.[1,10,11] These granulomas can be caseous and are generally composed of a central area of necrosis with accumulation of eosinophilic debris and surrounded by a layer of multinucleated giant cells (**Fig. 11**A).

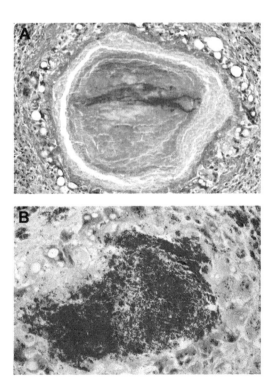

Fig. 11. Chicken (*Gallus gallus*), liver. (*A*) Photomicrograph of a typical granuloma with central necrosis and surrounding macrophages and giant cells (hematoxylin and eosin stain). (*B*) Same lesion as in *A* with numerous AFB in the center of the granuloma (Ziehl-Nielsen stain, original magnification ×20).

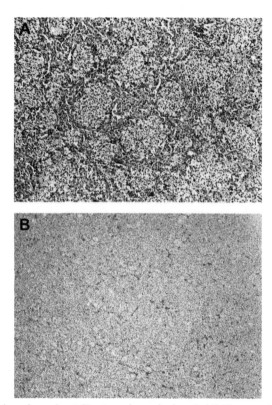

Fig. 12. Canary-winged parakeet (*Brotogeris versicolurus*). (*A*) Liver: multifocal aggregates of foamy macrophages without any evidence of necrosis (hematoxylin and eosin stain [H&E], original magnification ×20). (*B*) Spleen: sheets of foamy macrophages completely replacing the splenic tissue (H&E, original magnification ×10).

This in turn can be surrounded by macrophages or histiocytes, lymphocytes, and, occasionally, plasma cells and heterophils. In chronic stages of the disease, these granulomas can be surrounded by a layer of fibrous connective tissue. Acid-fast stain of these granulomas reveals numerous AFB within the central necrotic area but they can also be found in the cytoplasm of multinucleated giant cells and macrophages (see **Fig. 11**B).[1,10] Occasionally, multinucleated giant cells may not be present in the mycobacterial granulomas. There may also be overlapping of or variation in the nature of histologic lesions from bird to bird.

The most common type of histopathologic lesions in psittacines and passerines such as canaries and finches is infiltration of a large number of epithelioid cells or foamy macrophages, with or without multinucleated giant cells but lacking tissue necrosis (**Fig. 12**).[3,8,50,51,71] This type of histologic reaction resembles lesions seen in leprosy and as such has been called "lepromatous reaction." The macrophages are usually arranged as aggregates or sheets and are uniformly large with faintly staining bluish cytoplasm filled with faintly staining rod-shaped bacilli.[6] With a lack of experience in recognizing such lesions and without acid-fast staining of the lesions, the reaction can be confused for some form of neoplasia. The cytoplasm of giant cells is also blue and contains faintly staining rod-shaped bacilli.[6] The severe infiltration of such macrophages in the lamina propria of the intestine accounts for the numerous

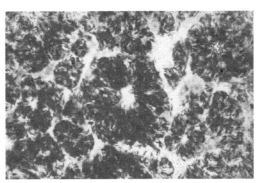

Fig. 13. Canary-winged parakeet (*Brotogeris versicolurus*). Photomicrograph of the spleen showing numerous acid-fast bacteria in the cytoplasm of macrophages (Ziehl-Nielsen stain, original magnification ×100).

miliary nodules seen grossly in the mucosa of the intestine.[63] Acid-fast staining of such lesions reveals myriads of AFB in the cytoplasm of macrophages and giant cells (**Fig. 13**).

The second type of inflammatory reaction less commonly seen in psittacines is similar to the above-described reaction except that there is infiltration of lymphocytes and, rarely, plasma cells and heterophils at the periphery of the macrophage aggregates, especially in the liver.[4] The third type of reaction, which is not common in psittacines, is similar to the reaction seen in gallinaceous birds and was observed only in the air sacs and peritoneum.[54] There may be variation in or overlapping of these 3 types of histologic lesions from bird to bird.

SUMMARY

Avian mycobacteriosis is an important and common disease that affects companion, captive exotic, wild, and domestic birds. The disease in birds is generally caused by *M avium* subsp *avium*, but more than 10 other species of mycobacteria have been known to infect birds. Mycobacteriosis due to *M genavense* is more common in psittacines and passerines such as canaries and finches. Oral route of infection appears to be the primary mode of transmission of mycobacteriosis in birds based on the lesions most commonly found in the intestine and liver. In some cases, the extensive involvement of the respiratory system, especially the lungs, suggests an airborne mode of transmission. Gross lesions due to mycobacteriosis range from enlargement and the presence of pale-yellow nodules in the liver, spleen, intestine, bone marrow, and other organs and histologic lesions of granulomas composed of necrosis and multinucleated giant cells, macrophages, and other inflammatory cells in gallinaceous birds, raptors, and wild birds to diffuse enlargement and pale mottling of the liver and spleen and military nodules in the intestine and histologic lesions composed of macrophages and giant cell infiltration in psittacines. Acid-fast staining reveals numerous AFB in the cytoplasm of macrophages and giant cells. In the past years, molecular diagnostic techniques have improved the ability to confirm the disease suspected by gross and histopathologic examination, aiding in rapid identification and characterization of *Mycobacterium* subsp, overcoming the disadvantages of conventional methods. Avian mycobacteriosis should not be underestimated since it represents an important veterinary and economic risk in birds as well as mammals. Exposure of humans to infected birds may cause a zoonotic infection, especially in those with immunocompromising diseases.

REFERENCES

1. Montali RJ, Busch M, Theon CO, et al. Tuberculosis in captive exotic birds. J Am Vet Med Assoc 1976;169:920–7.
2. Keymer IF, Jones DM, Pugsley SL, et al. A survey of tuberculosis in birds in the Regent's Park gardens of the Zoological Society of London. Avian Pathol 1982;11: 563–9.
3. Gerlach H. Bacteria. In: Ritchie B, Harrison G, Harrison L, eds. Avian medicine, principles and application. Lake Worth (FL): Wingers Publishing; 1994. p. 949–83.
4. Hoop RK, Böttger EC, Pfyffer GE. Etiological agents of mycobacteriosis in pet birds between 1986 and 1995. J Clin Microbiol 1996;34:991–2.
5. Thoen CO, Richards WD, Jarnagin JL. Mycobacteria isolated from exotic animals. J Am Vet Med Assoc 1977;170:987–90.
6. Tell LA, Woods L, Cromie RL. Mycobacteriosis in birds. Rev Sci Tech 2001;20:180–203.
7. Lennox AM. Mycobacteriosis in companion psittacine birds: a review. J Avian Med Surg 2007;21:181–7.
8. Manarolla G, Liandris E, Pisoni G, et al. Mycobacterium genavense and avian polyomavirus co-infection in a European goldfinch (Carduelis carduelis). Avian Pathol 2007;36:423–6.
9. Heatley JJ, Mitchell MM, Roy A, et al. Disseminated mycobacteriosis in a bald eagle. J Avian Med Surg 2007;21:201–9.
10. Fulton RM, Sanchez S. Tuberculosis. In: Saif YM, Fadly AM, Glisson JR, et al, editors. Diseases of poultry. 12th edition. Ames (IO): Iowa Blackwell; 2008.
11. Milla J, Negre N, Castalenos E, et al. Avian mycobacteriosis in free-living raptors in Majorca Island, Spain. Avian Pathol 2010;9:1–6.
12. Antinoff N, Kiehn TE, Bottger EC. Mycobacteriosis caused by Mycobacterium genavense in a psittacine bird. Proc Annu Conf Assoc Avian Vet 1996;169–70.
13. Bercovier H, Vincent V. Mycobacterial infections in domestic and wild animals due to Mycobacterium marinum, M. fortuitum, M. chelonae, M. porcinum, M. farcinogenes, M. smegmatis, M. scrofulaceum, M. xenopi, M. kansasii, M. simiae and M. genavense. Rev Sci Tech 2001;20:265–90.
14. Bertelsen MF, Grøndahl C, Giese SB. Disseminated Mycobacterium celatum infection in a white-tailed trogon (Trogon viridis). Avian Pathol 2006;35:316–9.
15. Holsboer Buogo C, Bacciarini L, et al. Occurrence of Mycobacterium genavense in birds. Schweiz Arch Tierheilkd 1997;139:397–402.
16. Hoop RK, Böttger EC, Ossent P, et al. Mycobacteriosis due to Mycobacterium genavense in six pet birds. J Clin Microbiol 1993;31:990–3.
17. Kik MJ, Houwers DJ, Dinkla A. Mycobacterium intermedium granulomatous pneumonia in a green oropendola (Psarocolius viridis). Vet Rec 2010;167: 219–20.
18. Ledwon A, Szeleszczuk P, Malicka E, et al. Mycobacteriosis caused by Mycobacterium genavense in lineolated parakeets (Bolborhynchus lineola). A case report. Bull Vet Inst Pulawy 2009;53:209–12.
19. Miranda A, Pires MA, Pinto ML, et al. Mycobacterium avium subspecies paratuberculosis in a diamante sparrow. Vet Rec 2009;165:184.
20. Montali RJ, Mikota SK, Cheng LI. Mycobacterium tuberculosis in zoo and wildlife species. Rev Sci Tech 2001;20:291–303.

21. Portaels F, Realini L, Bauwens L, et al. *Mycobacterium genavense* in birds kept in a zoo: 11-year survey. J Clin Microbiol 1996;34:319–23.
22. Shitaye JE, Halouzka R, Svobodova J, et al. First isolation of *Mycobacterium genavense* in a blue headed parrot (*Pionus menstruus*) imported from Surinam (South America) to the Czech Republic: a case report. Vet Med 2010;55:339–47.
23. Travis EK, Junge RE, Terrell SP. Infection with Mycobacterium simiae complex in four captive Micronesian kingfishers. J Am Vet Med Assoc 2007;230:1524–9.
24. Vitali SD, Eden PA, Payne KL, et al. An outbreak of mycobacteriosis in Gouldian finches caused by Mycobacterium peregrinum. Vet Clin North Am Exot Anim Pract 2006;9(3):519–22.
25. Manarolla G, Liandris E, Pisoni G, et al. Avian mycobacteriosis in companion birds: 20-year survey. Vet Microbiol 2009;133:323–7.
26. Witte CL, Hungerford LL, Papendick R, et al. Investigation of characteristics and factors associated with mycobacteriosis in birds. J Vet Diagn Invest 2008;20:186–96.
27. Van der Heyden N. Mycobacteriosis. In: Rosskopf W, Woerpel R, editors. Diseases of cage and aviary birds. Baltimore (MD): Williams and Wilkins; 1996. p. 568–71.
28. Qureshi MA, Heggen CL, Hussain I. Avian macrophage: effector functions in health and disease. Dev Comp Immunol 2000;24:103–19.
29. Hines ME, Kreeger JM, Herron AJ. Mycobacterial infections of animals: pathology and pathogenesis. Lab Anim Sci 1995;45:334–51.
30. Rocco JM, Irani VR. Mycobacterium avium and modulation of the host macrophage immune mechanisms. Int J Tuberc Lung Dis 2011;15:447–52.
31. Sweet L, Singh PP, Azad AK, et al. Mannose receptor-dependent delay in phagosome maturation by *Mycobacterium avium* glicopeptidolipids. Infect Immun 2010;78:518–26.
32. Cheville NF, Richards WD. The influence of thymic and bursal lymphoid systems in avian tuberculosis. Am J Pathol 1971;64:97–122.
33. Dhama K, Mahendran M, Tiwari R, et al. Tuberculosis in Birds: Insights into the Mycobacterium avium Infections. Vet Med Int 2011. doi:10.4061/2011/712369.
34. Ackerman LJ, Benbrook SC, Walton BC. *Mycobacterium tuberculosis* infection in a parrot (*Amazona farinosa*). Am Rev Respir Dis 1974;109:388–90.
35. Brown R. Sinus, articular and subcutaneous *Mycobacterium tuberculosis* infection in a juvenile red-lored amazon parrot. Proc Annu Conf Assoc Avian Vet 1990;305–8.
36. Ferrer L, Ramis A, Fernandez J, et al. Granulomatous dermatitis caused by *Mycobacterium genavense* in two psittacine birds. Vet Derm 1997;8:213–9.
37. Hinshaw WR. Tuberculosis of human origin in the Amazon parrot. Am Rev Tuberc 1933;28:273–8.
38. Washko RM, Hoefer H, Kiehn TE, et al. *Mycobacterium tuberculosis* infection in a green-winged macaw (*Ara chloroptera*): report with public health implications. J Clin Microbiol 1998;36:1101–2.
39. Peters M, Proddinger WM, Gummer H, et al. *Mycobacterium tuberculosis* infection in a blue-fronted amazon parrot (*Amazona aestiva aestiva*). Vet Microbiol 2007;122:381–3.
40. Bowes V. Avian tuberculosis in ostriches. Can Vet J 1993;34:758.
41. Muller MG, George AR, Walochnik J. Acinetobacter baumannii in localized cutaneous mycobacteriosis in falcons. Vet Med Int 2010;2010.pii: ID321797.
42. Hoefer HL, Kiehn TE, Friedan TR. Systemic *Mycobacterium tuberculosis* in a green-winged macaw. Proc Annu Conf Assoc Avian Vet 1996:167–8.
43. Woerpel RW, Rosskopf WG. Retro-orbital *Mycobacterium tuberculosis* infection in a yellow-naped Amazon parrot (*Amazona ochracephala auropalliata*). Proc Annu Conf Assoc Avian Vet 1983:71–6.

44. Sevcikova Z, Ledecky V, Capik I, et al. Unusual manifestation of tuberculosis in ostrich (*Struthio camelus*). Vet Rec 1999;145:708.

45. Stanz KM, Miller PE, Cooley AJ, et al. Mycobacterial keratitis in a parrot. J Am Vet Med Assoc 1995;206(8):1177–80.

46. Gonzalez M, Rodriguez-Berros A, Gimeno I, et al. Outbreaks of avian tuberculosis in 48-week-old commercial layer hen flock. Avian Dis 2002;46:1055–61.

47. Steinmetz HW, Rutz C, Hoop RK, et al. Possible human-avian transmission of *Mycobacterium tuberculosis* in a green-winged macaw (*Ara chloroptera*). Avian Dis 2006;50:641–5.

48. Dolphin RE, Olsen DE, Gallina AM. Tubercular infection in a sulfur-crested cockatoo. Vet Med Small Anim Clin 1979;74:833–5.

49. Drew L, Ramsay E. Dermatitis associated with *Mycobacterium spp*. in a blue-fronted Amazon parrots. Proc Annu Conf Assoc Avian Vet 1991:252–3.

50. Saggese MD, Tizard I, Phalen DN. Mycobacteriosis in naturally infected ring-neck doves (Streptopelia risoria): investigation of the association between feather colour and susceptibility to infection, disease and lesions type. Avian Pathol 2008;37:443–50.

51. Saggese MD, Riggs G, Tizard I, et al. Gross and microscopic findings and investigation of the aetiopathogenesis of mycobacteriosis in a captive population of white-winged ducks (Cairina scutulata). Avian Pathol 2007;36:415–22.

52. Kock ND, Kock RA, Wambua J et al. *Mycobacterium avium* related epizootic in free ranging lesser flamingos in Kenya. J Wildl Dis 1999;35:297–300.

53. Sykes GP. Tuberculosis in a Red-Tailed Hawk (Buteo Jamaicensis). J Wildl Dis 1982;18:495–9.

54. Schmidt RE, Reavill DR, Phalen DN. Pathology of pet and aviary birds. Ames (IO): Blackwell; 2003.

55. Schmidt V, Schneider S, Schlomer J, et al. Transmission of tuberculosis between men and pet birds: a case report. Avian Pathol 2008;37:589–92.

56. Sousa E, Momo C, Costa TP, et al. Disseminated avian tuberculosis in captive Ara macao. Braz J Vet Pathol 2008;1:28–31.

57. Odiawo GO, Mukurira JM. Avian cerebral tuberculosis. Vet Rec 1988;122:279–80.

58. Forster F, Gerlach H. Mycobacteria in psittaciformes. Proc Annu Conf Assoc Avian Vet 1987:39–56.

59. Ramis A, Ferrer L, Aranaz A, et al. *Mycobacterium genavense* infection in canaries. Avian Dis 1996;40:246–51.

60. Britt GO, Howard EB, Rosskopf WG. Psittacine tuberculosis. Cornell Vet 1980;70: 218–25.

61. Butcher GD, Reed WM, Winterfield RW, Nilipour A. *Mycobacterium* infection in a gray-cheeked parakeet. Avian Dis 1990;34:1023–6.

62. Hoop RK, Ehrsam H, Ossent P, et al. Mycobacteriosis of ornamental birds: frequency, pathologo-anatomic, histologic and microbiologic data. Berl Munch Tierarztl Wochenschr 1994;107:275–81.

63. Shitaye EJ, Grymova V, Grym M, et al. *Mycobacterium avium subsp. hominissuis* infection in a pet parrot. Emerg Infect Dis 2009;15:617–9.

64. Mitchinson MJ, Keymer IF. Tuberculous aortitis in birds. J Comp Pathol 1972;82: 483–6.

65. Morton LD, Ehrhart EJ, Briggs MB, et al. Granulomatous aortitis and cardiopulmonary arteritis in fairy-bluebird (Irena puella) with mycobacteriosis. Proc Am Assoc Zoo Vet 1997;272–3.

66. Shivaprasad HL. Amyloidosis in commercial Pekin ducks. 35th Annual meeting of the American Association of Veterinary Laboratory Diagnosticians 1992;63.

67. Riddell C, Atkinson DR. Two cases of mycobacteriosis in psittacine birds. Can Vet J 1981;22:145–7.
68. Panigrahy B, Clark FD, Hall CF. Mycobacteriosis in psittacine birds. Avian Dis 1983;267:1166–8.
69. Tell LA, Woods L, Foley J, et al. A model of avian mycobacteriosis: clinical and histopathologic findings in Japanese quail (*Coturnix coturnix japonica*) intravenously inoculated with *Mycobacterium avium*. Avian Dis 2003;47:433–43.
70. Gomez G, Saggese M, Porter BF, et al. Granulomatous intestinal ganglioneuritis and encephalomyelitis in a spectacled Amazon parrot (*Amazona albifrons*) infected with *Mycobacterium genavense*. Comp Pathol 2011;144:219–22.
71. Rae MA, Rosskopf WJ. Mycobacteriosis in passerines. Proc Annu Conf Assoc Avian Vet 1992:234–43.

Taking a Rational Approach in the Treatment of Avian Mycobacteriosis

Jennifer Buur, DVM, PhD, DACVCP*, Miguel D. Saggese, DVM, MS, PhD

KEYWORDS

- *Mycobacterium* • Mycobacteriosis • Birds • Antibiotics
- Pharmacokinetics • Treatment

Mycobacterial infections threaten a wide range of species of pet birds, causing a typically chronic and debilitating and typically fatal disease usually referred to as mycobacteriosis.[1] Avian mycobacteriosis is in fact a group of different infectious diseases caused by several species of bacteria of the genus *Mycobacterium*. They all have in common a chronic, granulomatous pattern of inflammatory response as result of the immune system trying to contain and eliminate, most times unsuccessfully, the microorganism (see article by Shivaprasad and Palmieri elsewhere in this issue for further exploration of this topic). Many species of mycobacteria have been found to cause disease in birds, including *Mycobacterium avium* subsp *avium*, *M genavense*, *M tuberculosis*, *M simiae*, *M gordonae*, *M intracellulare*, *M intermedium*, *M peregrinum*, *M terrae*, *M avium* subsp *paratuberculosis*, *M avium* subsp *hominissuis*, *M trivial*, *M fortuitum*, *M diernhoferi*, *M chelonae*, *M smegmatis*, *M flavescens*, *M scrofulaceum*, and *M celatum*.[3] However, *M avium* subsp *avium* and *M genavense* account for most of the confirmed cases of mycobacteriosis in companion pet birds.[2–4] *Mycobacterium avium* subsp *avium* seems to be less common in psittacinae and songbirds as most recent reports incriminate *M genavense* as the etiological agent of mycobacteriosis in these species (see article by Mark D. Schrenzel elsewhere in this issue for further exploration of this topic).[2–4] Clinical presentation, pathogenesis, pathology, diagnosis, and epidemiologic aspects of avian mycobacteriosis are outside the scope of this article and have been described elsewhere (see articles by Shivaprasad and Palmieri, Mark D. Schrenzel, and Dahlhausen and colleagues elsewhere in this issue for further exploration of this topic).[2,5–14]

Important differences of opinion exist between avian practitioners and the avian medicine literature as to whether cases of avian mycobacteriosis should be treated.

The authors have nothing to disclose.

College of Veterinary Medicine, Western University of Health Sciences, 309 East Second Street, Pomona, CA 91766, USA

* Corresponding author.

E-mail address: jbuur@westernu.edu

vetexotic.theclinics.com

Box 1
Cognitive framework for the use of therapeutics

- Establishment of a diagnosis
- Evaluation of treatment options
- Evidence-based drug choice
- Optimized dosing regimen
- Establishment of treatment length
- Monitoring for treatment success and adverse effects
- Reflection on efficacy of treatment

Euthanasia is usually recommended[1,9,12,15–17] based on a perceived zoonotic risk of mycobacterial infections for the immunocompromised, children, and the elderly. Also, the lack of scientific research conducted on treatment of mycobacteriosis in birds precludes an evidence-based approach to the problem. Additional reasons in favor of euthanasia are the expensive and prolonged course of multidrug therapy that most mycobacterial infections are thought to require. Furthermore, the difficulty of drug administration to avian patients, natural and acquired antimicrobial drug resistance in many isolates, and poor owner compliance are additional reasons for euthanasia.[1,9,12] Arguments supporting the treatment of avian mycobacteriosis include the human–animal bond, economic value of individual birds, and conservation value of the affected bird or birds in a collection.[8,18–20] However, consensus about a rational approach to the treatment of mycobacteriosis in birds still is lacking.

The use of antimicrobial agents in the practice of veterinary medicine remains a cornerstone of treatment. In bacterial disease, it is often the only effective choice. However, as antibiotic resistance grows and the number of new drugs in development decreases, it becomes more important to have a thought framework (cognitive structure) on how to approach the use of these drugs. This rational and evidence-based approach has been developed in human medicine.[21] Similar strategies for veterinary drug therapies including antimicrobial use have been presented in the literature.[22] The overall process is presented in **Box 1**. Additionally, there is widespread use of therapy algorithms in human medicine when it comes to the treatment of bacterial disease. In veterinary medicine, guidelines for the safe and effective use of antimicrobials have been developed for use in companion animals, equine, aquatic animals, and food-producing species.[23–26] No set of guidelines has been developed for the treatment of bacterial disease in companion avian species. In human medicine, treatment of mycobacteriosis is both a medical and legal issue and treatment guidelines have been established and are often rigorously implemented (ie, observed compliance). In veterinary medicine, guidelines for the treatment of mycobacteriosis have been only established and implemented in elephants affected by tuberculosis (*M tuberculosis*), based on the human guidelines.[27] There is no reason that a rational approach could not be used in determining appropriate therapy and protocols in the treatment of avian mycobacteriosis. Therefore, the purpose of this article is to discuss an evidence-based approach to the treatment of mycobacteriosis in companion avian species using the framework presented in **Box 1**.

ESTABLISHMENT OF A DIAGNOSIS

Success of treatment is dependent on an accurate diagnosis and the precise identification of the bacterial organism (see article by Dahlhausen and colleagues elsewhere in this issue for further exploration of this topic). While it may not be appropriate to consider treatment in birds for species of Mycobacteria with well-recognized virulence and high zoonotic potential, such as M tuberculosis, with 33% of the world human population infected and a leading global cause of death,[28–30] treating birds with M avium subsp avium may pose a much lower risk to a bird's owner or caretaker. M avium isolates have been divided into 4 subspecies: M avium subsp avium, M avium subsp sylvaticum, M avium subsp paratuberculosis, and M avium subsp hominisuis.[31] These divisions are based on insertion sequence analysis, restriction fragment length polymorphism, and phenotypical and host differences. M avium subsp avium is considered as a separate taxon that affects birds and is differentiated from M avium subsp hominissuis, which affects pigs and humans (see article by Mark D. Schrenzel elsewhere in this issue for further exploration of this topic).[31] Recent studies suggest that the subspecies of M avium that commonly causes disease in immunocompromissed humans is Mycobacterium avium subsp hominissuis, not the subspecies that causes disease in birds (M avium subsp avium) (see article by Mark D. Schrenzel elsewhere in this issue for further exploration of this topic).[31–35] Despite this clear separation between human and avian isolates, mycobacteriosis caused by M avium subsp avium is still considered a potential zoonotic risk in the immunocompromised people, as occur with many other nontuberculous mycobacteria.

The other common species found in birds, M genavense (see articles by Shivaprasad and Palmieri, and Mark D. Schrenzel elsewhere in this issue for further exploration of this topic) is associated with gastrointestinal or pulmonary mycobacteriosis in HIV-positive or immunosuppressed human patients.[36,37] Only one report of M genavense infection exists in a healthy human.[38] M genavense is a slow-growing, environmental nontuberculous mycobacteria usually found in water. The infection seems to be rare in humans and no reports of this zoonosis can be found in the current literature.

Other species of mycobacteria less commonly reported in birds usually represent oportunistic infections, isolated cases, or specific outbreaks limited to single locations (see articles by Shivaprasad and Palmieri, and Mark D. Schrenzel elsewhere in this issue for further exploration of this topic).[39–43] Most species of mycobacteria reported in birds can potentially cause disease in humans as well, especially in the immunocompromised. The potential zoonotic risk can be easily determined if rapid and correct molecular characterization and identification of the species of mycobacteria affecting birds become an obligate step before attempting any treatment of these diseases in birds or any other exotic pet.

EVALUATION OF TREATMENT OPTIONS

While antimicrobial therapy is essential to the successful treatment of avian mycobacteriosis, husbandry remains an important adjunct treatment. Mycobacteria are resistant to many common disinfectants. Higher concentrations and longer contact times are necessary for optimum control. Alcohols, aldehydes, halogens, and phenolic agents are the most commonly used. Chlorohexidine and quaternary ammonium compounds (ie, bleach) are only mycobacteriostatic at best. Removal of all organic matter and other debris is essential to decrease the risk of self-reinfection

Table 1 Antimicrobial agents used in the treatment of mycobacteriosis[8,12,18,19,26,56]			
Antimicrobial Drug Class	Pharmacokinetic Studies Available in Avian Species	Optimal Dosing	Reported Use in the Treatment of Avian Mycobacteriosis (Refs.)
Isoniazid	No	Time dependent	Yes[8,19]
Rifamycin agents	Yes	Time dependent	Yes[18,19,26]
Pyrazinamide	No	Time dependent	Unknown
Ethambutol	No	Time dependent	Yes[8,19]
Aminoglycoside	Yes	Concentration dependent	Yes[18,19,26]
Fluoroquinolones	Yes	Concentration dependent	Yes[12,18,19]
Macrolides	Yes	Time dependent	Yes[8,19]
Ethionamide	No	Time dependent	Unknown
Cycloserine	No	Time dependent	Unknown
Aminosalicylic acid (PAS)	No	Time dependent	Unknown

and potential shed of mycobacteria exposed to antibiotics to other avian species, domestic animals, and humans.

Biosecurity measures should be implemented to help control possible spread of disease to other susceptible populations. Due to the zoonotic potential of these pathogens, limited exposure to humans is often advised. Those individuals with mycobacteriosis are recommended to be quarantined and removed from contact with other beyond the main caretaker as well from other birds, via both direct and indirect means, while under treatment.

There are very few published reports of attempts to treat affected birds. Such reports usually involve only a limited number of birds and consist mainly of clinical cases and case reports.[8,12,18,19,44] Most cases were reported before current molecular diagnostic techniques became readily available, thus preventing the exact identification of the species of Mycobacteria involved in the clinical case. In these reports, a wide range of antimicrobial agents, doses, and length of therapy have been recommended.[8,12,18,19,44] Dosing regimens were generally extrapolated from the human pediatric literature, calculated by metabolic allometrical scaling, or based on anecdotal reports.[8,12,18,19,44] More than 15 antimycobacterial drugs and combinations have been recommended to treat avian mycobacteriosis, although their efficacy is unknown given the lack of scientific research, both experimental and clinical (Table 1).

Successful treatment in birds may depend on the organism's susceptibility to the antibiotics, extent and localization of infection, and the immune response of the patient. These factors have not been fully determined before starting therapy in the reported cases of avian mycobacteriosis treatment.[8,18,19,39] Furthermore, the systemic presentation of the disease, most commonly affecting liver, spleen, intestines, and lungs, makes the clinical categorization of these patients difficult and thus limits our ability to compare treatment outcomes. Measures of treatment success have been judged by the improvement or resolution of clinical signs, the absence of acid-fast organisms and negative cultures, and/or polymerase chain reaction (PCR)-based assay of liver biopsies obtained at the end of treatment.[8,12,18,19,39,45] Nevertheless, liver biopsy and clinical improvement as measure of treatment efficacy are not a reliable evaluation of elimination of the infection status or of the health of the avian patient (see article by Dahlhausen and colleagues elsewhere in this issue for further exploration of this topic).[14] Mycobacteriosis caused by *M avium* subsp *avium* and *M genavense* have a multisystemic presentation in birds. Liver, spleen, bone marrow, and intestines are typically the main organs affected. While liver samples can be obtained by surgical or laparoscopic biopsy, they provide no information about the presence of lesions or mycobacteria in other organs. The finding of mycobacteria-free liver sections in naturally infected ring-neck doves that were positive in spleen and other organs raises concern about the sensitivity of using a single organ like the liver to evaluate treatment.[14] Detailed physical and clinical examination of the patient and investigation of multiple tissues and the use of several different diagnostic techniques may be a better form to evaluate response to antimycobacterial therapy in exotic pet birds (see article by Dahlhausen and colleagues elsewhere in this issue for further exploration of this topic).[14]

EVIDENCE-BASED DRUG CHOICE AND OPTIMIZED DOSING REGIMENS

With a high rate of mutation, mycobacteria develop resistance to antimicrobial agents at an alarming rate.[28,46] As a result of early observed single drug resistance, standard care in the treatment of humans with tuberculosis includes a multidrug regimen of a minimum of 3 or 4 different antibiotic drugs to prevent the emergence of antibiotic-resistant strains of mycobacteria.[28,46] In veterinary medicine, the only set protocols have been published for elephants with *M tuberculosis* infection.[27] These protocols include the use of 3 first-line agents in the first phase of treatment. Culture and sensitivity analysis should be used to determine which combination would provide the best efficacy for the specific individual. In the absence of this information, empirical treatment of respiratory disease in mammals would include a minimum of 3 or 4 first-line agents. However, since avian disease does not parallel tuberculosis in elephants, this type of empirical therapy cannot be recommended.

With the emergence of multidrug-resistant mycobacteriosis (MDR-TB; defined as bacteria resistant to at least isoniazid and rifampicin) and extremely drug-resistant mycobacteriosis (XDR-TB; defined as resistant to any fluoroquinolone and at least 1 of 3 injectable second-line drugs [capreomycin, kanamycin, and amikacin], in addition to being multidrug-resistant), it is has become even more important to use rational therapies with measurable outcomes. Nontuberculous *Mycobacteria* are particularly more naturally resistant to antimicrobial drugs than is *M tuberculosis.*[47,48] For the most part, the drugs and drug classes involved are not commonly used in veterinary medicine and may represent a large financial burden to the client depending on the size of the patient. Recommendations are generally extrapolated on human treatment regimens based on known pharmacokinetics of these agents in humans, in laboratory animals, and, in a few cases, when known, in birds. With limited exceptions, such as azithromycin and fluoroquinolones,[49,50] pharmacokinetic studies of antimycobacterial drugs in birds are lacking. These studies would be indispensable for a rational approach to the treatment of avian mycobacteriosis.[51] While the whole spectrum of avian patients probably cannot be covered, future studies on representative, highly susceptible, and most commonly kept pet species of Passeriformes, Psittaciformes, Columbiformes, Galliformes and Anseriformes are recommended given the higher prevalence of mycobacterial infections in these orders and they are all commonly kept as companion pet birds.

Drugs that are considered to be first-line agents in human medicine against tuberculosis (*M tuberculosis*) include isoniazid, rifampin or other rifamycin agents, pyrazinamide, ethambutol, and streptomycin.[28,46] Each of these agents has proven efficacy against *M tuberculosis* and often target different phases of replication and various antimicrobial targets. This increases the chance of sensitivity to at least part of the regimen even in the face of constant mutation. Second-line agents are used in humans when patients either stop responding to treatment clinically, culture and sensitivity reveal resistance to a first-line agent, or adverse effects limit the possibility of use.[28,46] Second-line agents include fluoroquinolones, other aminoglycosides, macrolides, ethionamide, aminosalicylic acid, cycloserine, and capreomycin.[28,46]

Given that nontuberculous mycobacterial infection in humans is a common problem in patients with AIDS and their sensitivity to antimyocbacterial drugs differs from *M tuberculosis*, treatment regimens using one of the new macrolide antibiotics, azithromycin or clarithromycin, in combination with ethambutol and rifampicines (rifampin or rifabutine) appears to be more effective in the treatment of *M avium* infection in patients with AIDS than older combinations of drugs.[52–54] Accordingly, a similar protocol has therefore been recommended for birds with mycobacteriosis.[8,12,18,19,44] However, the efficacy of these recommended protocols for treatment of *M avium* subsp *avium* is completely unknown.

In humans with *M genavense* infection, the recommended treatment includes a combination of streptomycin and rifampicin. This microorganism has been reported to be resistant in vitro to isoniazid and ethambutol. Other reported treatment of *M genavense* infection in human cases include combinations of moxifloxacin, clarythromycin, ethambutol, and amikacin[36–38]; however, the optimal treatment for *M genavense* infection in humans still is unknown.[55]

Pharmacokinetic studies and efficacy studies are lacking for most drugs and drug classes used in the treatment of avian tuberculosis. Dosing regimens for those drugs with pharmacokinetic data should be determined based on cultured minimum inhibitory concentrations (MIC) and appropriate pharmacokinetic-pharmacodynamic links. Doses for concentration-dependent drug classes should be optimized such that peak plasma drug concentration is 10 times the MIC of the pathogen or the area under the plasma concentration-time curve is 125 to 250 times the MIC. Time-dependent drug classes should be optimized such that plasma drug concentrations remain above the MIC for 90% of the dosing interval. Most commonly used antimycobacterial drugs are discussed next.[56]

Aminoglycosides

Aminoglycosides irreversibly bind to the 30S subunit of the bacterial ribosome leading to bactericidal activity. This class has a well-defined post antibiotic effect that can be maximized for greater efficacy while reducing the chance for toxicity. Toxicity occurs from interactions of aminoglycosides with specific phospholipids that result in pinocytosis and active uptake of the drug into the cells. Proximal renal tubular and cochlear cells have increased amounts of the phospholipid needed for uptake. Thus, renal, aural, and vestibular toxicity are the primary manifestations in exotic species. Streptomycin is the most common drug of this class used in the treatment of mycobacteriosis; it is considered to be a first-line drug in human medicine and is recommended as a possible first-line drug when treating elephants with *M tuberculosis* infection. Other aminoglycosides such as amikacin are generally considered to be second-line drugs. There are no reports of aminoglycoside use for mycobacteriosis in any exotic species, and its use in birds has been limited. Aminoglycosides are concentration-dependent antimicrobial agents. Toxicity is limited when the dosing interval is extended such that trough plasma concentrations are zero.

Fluoroquinolones

Moxifloxacin is the most commonly used fluoroquinolone in human medicine for tubercular mycobacteriosis and nontuberculous mycobacteria infections. In exotic species, enrofloxacin has been largely used in combination with other therapeutics. All fluoroquinolones inhibit topoisomerases including DNA gyrase and thus inhibit the unwinding of DNA during replication. Fluoroquinolones are one of the few groups of antibiotics with pharmacokinetics studies available for birds and other exotic species. These drugs are concentration dependent and are used widely in exotic animal medicine for other diseases. Toxicity from this drug class is relatively minor and consists of cartilage damage in growing animals and retinal degeneration in cats.

Macrolides

Macrolide antimicrobial agents (erythromycin, tulathromycin, tilmicosin, tylosin, clarithromycin, azithromycin) have been used successfully to treat multiple infectious diseases in a wide variety of exotic species. These drugs bind to the bacterial 50S ribosome and inhibit the lengthening of the protein chain by inhibiting the translocation of tRNA from the amino acid receptor site. While generally considered to be bacteriostatic, this drug class can have weak bactericidal activity depending on the specific strain involved. They work in a time-dependent manner. Antimicrobial activity is reduced in acidic environments including the microenvironment of tubercular mycobacteriosis. Azithromycin is a drug frequently used in the treatment of several nontuberculous mycobacterial infections in humans. Tissue concentrations of macrolides are generally higher than plasma concentrations. This has been demonstrated in tissues such as lung, liver, spleen, kidneys, and various body fluids including prostatic fluid and bile. Toxicity of macrolides is generally gastrointestinal in nature. Tilmicosin is the exception as it targets the heart by depleting intracellular calcium, leading to a negative inotropic effect. Accidental exposure in humans has resulted in multiple deaths. Similar toxicity has been established in horses, goats, pigs, and nonhuman primates. Tilmicosin in not recommended for use in the treatment of mycobacteriosis.

Rifamycins

Of the multiple rifamycins available, rifampin remains the most common drug used in veterinary medicine. Rifampin has good activity against many gram-positive microbes including most species of *Mycobacterium*. Rifamycins inhibit RNA chain initiation through inactivation of the DNA-dependent RNA polymerases. Efficacy is time dependent. At low concentrations, rifamycins are bacteriostatic. However, bactericidal concentrations are achieved in humans using standard tuberculosis dosing regimens. Rifampin, in particular, has been demonstrated to have synergistic effects with streptomycin and isoniazid in vitro against *M tuberculosis*. Resistance to rifamycin occurs through a single step that alters the confirmation of the DNA-dependent RNA polymerase leading to decreased drug binding. Rifampin induces cytochrome P450 enzymes as well as the P-glycoprotein pump leading to increased metabolism and decreased oral absorption of P450 and P-glycoprotein substrates respectively. The most common adverse effect is hepatitis. Urine, saliva, and tears can turn red-orange. Rifampin has been reported to be teratogenic. The pharmacokinetics of rifampin has not been reported in exotic pet birds.

Ethambutol

Ethambutol is a bacteriostatic drug with specific antibacterial activity against *M tuberculosis, M kansasii*, and *M avium* strains only. Ethambutol's activity is related to inhibition of arabinosyl transferases, which are important in cell wall synthesis, and activity is time dependent. Pharmacokinetic studies have only been published for mammals. Toxicities in humans include optic neuritis, hypersensitivities, and gastrointestinal upset. Increased blood urate concentrations occur in about half of all human patients. This may have significance when using ethambutol in avian species given their altered urate metabolism. Monitoring urate levels is recommended in all patients.

Isoniazid

Isoniazid is a mainstay of treatment in human disease. This is a prodrug that must be metabolized by bacterial enzymes into a potent inhibitor of mycolic acid production. Mycolic acids, besides being unique to this microbial species, are structural portions of the cell wall. Inhibition leads to rapid bactericidal effects when the organisms are in a growing phase. Little to no effect is derived when the bacteria has entered into "latency." This drug should not be given with other drugs that are bacteriostatic in nature. Dosing should be implemented assuming time-dependent activity. Resistance to isoniazid occurs rapidly in vivo. Treatment should include multiple drugs to help slow the development of resistance. No data are available to evaluate the effectiveness or pharmacokinetics of this drug in avian species.

Pyrazinamide

Pyrazinamide is bactericidal through alterations of the mycobacterial fatty acid synthase I gene. This gene is essential for mycolic acid biosythnesis and thus alters cell wall permeability. Resistance develops quickly in monotherapy conditions. Activity of pyrazinamide is increased in acidic environments such as the phagosome of macrophages (a common site of mycobacterium infections). Activity is assumed to be time dependent. No information is available for use in birds.

ESTABLISHMENT OF TREATMENT LENGTH

Treatment of mycobacteriosis is complicated regardless of the species. The organisms are intracellular and not only grow slowly but also have high rates of mutation to key antimicrobial targets. However, the success in treatment of human beings can provide some insight into the treatment of avian species. It is important to note that the most common form of mycobacteriosis in humans is tubercular in nature. This form has been reported in birds (see article by Shivaprasad and Palmieri elsewhere in this issue for further exploration of this topic). Atypical or nontubercular mycobacteriosis requires different strategies for maximal therapeutic efficacy including alternate drug choices and different dosing regimens.

An important consideration of antimicrobial therapy is length of treatment. Since most pathogenic mycobacteria are slow-growing microorganisms that can go into "latency" states, therapy is prolonged and can last for years.[28] In humans affected with the tuberculous bacilli, the World Health Organization recommends an initial phase lasting 3 months with subsequent phases lasting up to 2 years. While human medicine can initiate directly observed therapy to ensure compliance, this remains outside of the realm for most veterinary practices, generating an additional challenge.

For the veterinary professional, the extended length of treatment provides some unique challenges. Many species will refuse medications when given over a prolonged period of time or will become extremely aggressive after the permanent stress of handling them. For private parties, this decreases the human–animal bond and can lead to poor compliance. Owner and handler compliance becomes vastly more important when it is realized that drug resistance increases several fold for every dose missed. Finally, it is unknown what adverse effects may occur due to prolonged treatment in avian species. Clearly there is work to be done on this topic. More research on simple, nonforced, effective, and economic forms of long-term drug administration in companion pet birds, particularly on species difficult to medicate orally such as Psittaciformes and small Passeriformes, is needed for the potential implementation of any antimycobacterial therapy.

MONITORING FOR TREATMENT SUCCESS AND ADVERSE EFFECTS

Another important and uninvestigated area in birds receiving treatment includes the natural or acquired drug resistance observed in most species of mycobacteria, particularly *M avium* subsp *avium* and *M genavense*. Development of drug resistance is a common complication of treatment of humans with mycobacterial infections, especially for tuberculosis (*M tuberculosis*) and nontuberculous mycobacteria such as *M avium* subsp *hominissuis*.[52,53] Multidrug treatment is necessary to prevent the selection of drug-resistant mutants during therapy. Most isolates of *M avium* complex have naturally and acquired resistance to many antimycobacterial drugs.[53–55] Development of antibiotic resistance has not yet been investigated in birds with mycobacteriosis before and after therapy. In humans, development of drug resistance usually occurs due to lack of compliance, so the same commitment and compliance of the owner regarding treatment of avian pets are essential for a successful outcome. In humans, multidrug resistance is an increasing and emerging problem for the treatment of tuberculosis and other human mycobacteriosis,[57] and given the zoonotic risk of mycobacterial infections, it is essential to investigate the possible presence of natural and/or acquired drug resistance in avian clinical isolates. Limitations to the investigation of drug resistance by classic microbiological methods are the long turnaround time required to culture *M avium* and particularly *M genavense*. The antimicrobial susceptibility testing is also not fully standardized for some drugs and nontuberculous mycobacteria. Recently, the use of PCR for the amplification and identification of antibiotic resistance genes has been gaining increased attention.[58–60] Drug resistance patterns can be identified by molecular methods directly from mycobacteria present in exudates or affected biopsied tissues sampled by laparoscopy, endoscopy, celiotomy, and fine needle aspiration. This can be done in a much shorter period of time (days) and can be performed by several molecular diagnostic laboratories. An important advantage of this method is the rapid turnaround time. Concurrent species, subspecies, and even strain identification and antimicrobial resistance patterns can be now obtained in less than 24 hours. Again, further research is needed on this new available technique for their direct application on avian myobacteriosis.

Isolates from birds with mycobacteriosis should be tested before and after treatment for the presence of antibiotic resistance genes. Primary natural antibiotic resistance genes and gene mutations associated with this acquired resistance are available for some species of *Mycobacteria* like *M tuberculosis* and *M avium* isolates from humans.[61,62] For example, the use of PCR for the investigation of 23S rRNA mutations in MAC isolates has proved useful for rapid detection of clarithromycin resistance.[62] Primers and PCR parameters used for amplification and sequencing of these genes involved in resistance have been published elsewhere.[58–60,63] Concurrent examination with conventional antibiotic sensitivity tests (available at The National Jewish Medical and Research Center, Colorado) should be performed and when available compared with molecular results. As it occurs with many other antibiotics in vitro and in vivo sensitivity/resistance patterns do not always correlate.

The chronicity of treatment makes these cases ideal for therapeutic drug monitoring. Many of the therapeutics involved induce P450 enzymes and can alter the metabolism of themselves and others.[56] In elephants, therapeutic drug monitoring is essential to prove adequate treatment.[27] Drug levels should be based on culture results, although this is essentially difficult in the case of mycobacteria given their prolonged culturing time. Absorption can be variable depending on a wide variety of factors including formulation, food intake, and gastric motility. Furthermore, mycobacteriosis in birds usually affects intestine and liver and moderate to severe malfunctioning of these organs, interfering with normal absorption and metabolism of these drugs. Ideally, both peak and trough samples should be submitted for drug quantification. However, this is often impractical given the size and stress of handling in avian patients. As a rule of thumb, peak samples are more important for concentration dependent drugs while trough samples are more valuable for time-dependent drugs. Finally, the long-term use of any therapeutic requires consistent monitoring of general patient health. All patients should be routinely screened for evidence of hepatic or renal dysfunction.

SUMMARY AND FUTURE DIRECTIONS

Treatment for avian mycobacteriosis is still in its infancy based on extrapolations from human medicine. The optimum drug choice, dose, or length of treatment has yet to be determined for most exotic animal species. Treatment should include multiple drugs for extended periods of time with appropriate monitoring of both drug levels and overall animal health. Risk to owners and handlers needs to be minimized through appropriate identification of the species of mycobacteri causing disease. Furthermore, more research needs to be done on the pharmacokinetics of these drugs in other animal species and antibiotic resistance. Currently, euthanasia remains the most common action in the face of active mycobacteriosis.

Rational treatment of avian mycobacteriosis is possible. However, the literature suggests that there is not enough evidence-based and scientific knowledge to effectively treat the avian patient with antimycobacterial drugs. Consistent, multidisciplinary, coordinated, and collaborative research is therefore needed before treatment of mycobacteriosis in birds should be pursued in avian medicine practice.

The following conclusions summarize some recommendations, and future direction that could be the starting point to effectively undertake the challenges associated with the treatment of mycobacterial infections in birds. The authors advocate for the adherence to these guidelines and recommendations and do not recommend at this time the medical treatment of any exotic pet bird affected with mycobacteriosis. At the same time, we propose the creation of a panel of experts to further discuss these concepts and recommendations through a consensual approach in the frame of evidence-based medicine.

- Research on avian mycobacteriosis treatment should focus, at least initially, on the 2 most common agents responsible of the majority of avian mycobacteriosis cases: *M avium* subsp *avium* and *M genavense*. These are the 2 more prevalent mycobacteria found in companion birds. Reports of other species of mycobacteria in birds usually are single and localized and possibly are not prioritary for research compared with these other 2 microorganisms.
- Companion pet parrots, pigeons, songbirds, pet chickens, and waterfowl are highly susceptible to avian mycobacteriosis. Emphasis on pharmacokinetics

studies of antimycobacterial drugs and drug administration should be put on these avian species first.

- Pharmacokinetic studies for drugs with known in vitro efficacy need to be performed to determine rational doses for use in avian mycobacteriosis. These studies would be followed by clinical trials in both experimental and field environments.
- An exhaustive diagnostic approach and clinical categorization of affected individuals potentially used in clinical trials and research should be followed. A classification of clinical stages of mycobacteriosis is not available at this time.
- Antibiotic susceptibility and resistance in avian isolates of mycobacteria should be investigated by molecular methods. This is an area that has not been addressed in avian medicine. Concurrent antibiotic susceptibility by classic microbiological methods should be pursued. Post-treatment, independent of the outcome, investigation of acquired antibiotic resistance is further recommended to assess the potential development of multidrug resistant strains of mycobacteria.
- The immune response to mycobacteriosis in exotic pet birds is poorly known and progress in this field is needed as mycobacteriosis usually appears to occur as result of an undermined immune system.

The end result of these collaborative efforts would be the creation of treatment guidelines for the avian practitioner. We are confident that safe, effective treatment options can be created using the tenets of evidence-based medicine. Rational treatment of avian mycobacteriosis is within our grasp.

REFERENCES

1. Tell L, Woods L, Cromie RL. Mycobacteriosis in birds. Rev Sci Tech 2001;1:180–203.
2. Portaels F, Realini L, Bauwens LW. Mycobacteriosis caused by *Mycobacterium genavense* in birds kept in a zoo: 11-year study. J Clin Microbiol 1996;34:319–23.
3. Shivaprasad HL, Roy P, Dhillon AS. Mycobacteriosis in psittacines. Proceedings of the Association of Avian Veterinarians. Monterrey (CA), 2005. p.153–5
4. Manarolla G, Liandris E, Pisoni G, et al. Avian mycobacteriosis in companion birds: 20-year survey. Vet Microbiol 2009;133:323–7.
5. Cromie RL. A comparison and evaluation of techniques for diagnosis of avian tuberculosis in wildfowl. Avian Pathol 1993;22:617–30.
6. Cromie RL, Ash NJ, Brown MJ, et al. Avian immune response to Mycobacterium avium: the wildfowl example. Dev Comp Immunol 2000;24:169–85.
7. Aranaz A, Liébana E, Mateos A, et al. Laboratory diagnosis of avian mycobacteria. Semin Avian Exot Pet Med 1997;6:9–17.
8. Van Der Heyden N. Clinical manifestations of mycobacteriosis in pet birds. Semin Avian Exot Pet Med 1997;6:18–24.
9. Gerlach H. Bacteria. In: Ritchie BW, Harrison GJ, Harrison LR, editors. Avian medicine: principles and application. Gerlach (FL): Wingers Publishing; 2000. p. 949–83.
10. Tell LA, Foley J, Needham ML, et al. Diagnosis of avian mycobacteriosis: comparison of culture, acid fast stains, and polymerase chain reaction for the identification of *Mycobacterium avium* in experimentally inoculated Japanese quail (*Coturnix coturnix japonica*). Avian Dis 2003;47:444–52.
11. Schmidt RE, Reavill DR, Phalen D. Pathology of pet and aviary birds. Ames (IO): Blackwell Publishing, Iowa State Press; 2003.

12. Pollock CG. Implications of mycobacteria in clinical disorders. In: Harrison G, Lightfoot T, editors. Clinical avian medicine. Florida: Spix Publisher; 2006. p. 681–90.
13. Schrenzel M, Nicolas M, Witte C, et al. Molecular epidemiology of *Mycobacterium avium* subsp *avium* and *Mycobacterium intracellulare* in captive birds. Vet Microbiol 2008;126:122–31.
14. Saggese MD, Tizard I, Phalen DN. Comparison of sampling methods, culture, acid-fast stain, and polymerase chain reaction assay for the diagnosis of mycobacteriosis in ring-neck doves (*Streptopelia risoria*). J Avian Med Surg 2010:24:263–71.
15. Dorrestein GM. Infections caused by bacteria. In: Altman RB, Clubb SI, Dorrestein GM, et al, editors. Avian medicine and surgery. New York: WB Saunders; 1996.
16. Beynon PH, Forbes NA, Harcourt-Brown NH. BSAVA manual of pigeons, raptors and waterfowl. Cheltenham (UK): BSAVA Publishing; 1996.
17. Samour J. Avian medicine. New York: Mosby-Elsevier; 2008.
18. Lennox AM. Successful treatment of mycobacterial in three psittacine birds. Proceedings of the Association of Avian Veterinarians Annual Conference. Reno (NV), 2002. p. 111–4.
19. Lennox AM. Mycobacteriosis in companion psittacine birds: a review. J Avian Med Surg 2007:21:181–7.
20. Riggs G. Mycobacterial infection in waterfowl collections: a conservation perspective 2005. Proceedings of the Association of Avian Veterinarians Annual Conference. Monterey (CA), 2005. p. 70–6.
21. Bajcar J, Kennie N, Iglar K. Teaching pharmacotherapeutics to family medicine residents: a curriculum. Can Fam Physician 2008;54:549.
22. AVMA. Judicious therapeutic use of antimicrobials (oversight: FSAC; approved by the AVMA executive board, November 1998; revised April 2004, November 2008). Available at: http://www.avma.org/issues/policy/jtua.asp accessed 12/1/2011. Accessed November 12, 2011.
23. Anonymous. Judicious use of antimicrobials for treatment of aquatic animals by veterinarians (oversight: AqVMC; EB approved November 2002; revised November 2008) Available at: http://www.avma.org/reference/jtua.asp. Accessed November 12, 2011.
24. Anonymous. American Association of Feline Practitioners/American Animal Hospital Association basic guidelines of judicious therapeutic use of antimicrobials (approved by the AVMA executive board November 2006, revised April 2009). Available at: http://www.avma.org/reference/jtua.asp. Accessed November 12, 2011.
25. Anonymous. American Association of Equine Practitioners prudent drug usage guidelines (approved by the AVMA executive board June 2001). Available at: http://www.avma.org/reference/jtua.asp. Accessed November 12, 2011.
26. Anonymous. Approval and availability of antimicrobials for use in food producing animals (oversight: FSAC; proposed SCAR-03/03; approved EB-05/03; revised November 2008). Available at: http://www.avma.org/reference/jtua.asp. Accessed November 12, 2011.
27. Anonymous. Guidelines for the control of tuberculosis in elephants. The National Tuberculosis Working Group for Zoo and Wildlife Species. Available at: http://www.aphis.usda.gov/animal_welfare/downloads/elephant/elephant_tb.pdf. Accessed October 29, 2008.
28. Cole ST, Eisenach KD, McMurray DN, et al. Tuberculosis and the tubercle bacillus. Washington (DC): ASM Press; 2004.
29. Schmidt V, Schneider S, Schlomer J, et al. Transmission of tuberculosis between men and pet birds: a case report. Avian Pathol 2008;37:589–92.

30. Steinmetz HW, Rutz C, Hoop RK, et al. Possible human-avian transmission of *Mycobacterium tuberculosis* in a green-winged macaw (*Ara chloroptera*). Avian Dis 2006;50:641–5.
31. Mijs W, de Haas P, Rossau R, et al. Molecular evidence to support a proposal to reserve the designation *Mycobacterium avium* subsp *avium* for bird-type isolates and *M avium* subsp *hominissuis* for the human/porcine type of *M avium*. Int J Syst Evol Microbiol 2002:52(Pt 5):1505–18.
32. Pavlik I, Svastova P, Bartl J, et al. Relationship between IS901 in the Mycobacterium avium complex strains isolated from birds, animals, humans and environment and virulence for poultry. Clin Diagn Lab Immunol 2000;7:212–7.
33. Möbius P, Lentzsch P, Moser I, et al. Comparative macrorestriction and RFLP analysis of Mycobacterium avium subsp avium and Mycobacterium avium subsp hominissuis isolates from man, pig, and cattle. Vet Microbiol 2006;117:284–91.
34. Johansen TB, Olsen I, Jensen MR, et al. New probes used for IS1245 and IS1311 restriction fragment length polymorphism of *Mycobacterium avium* subsp *avium* and *Mycobacterium avium* subsp *hominissuis* isolates of human and animal origin in Norway. BMC Microbiol 2007;5:7–14.
35. Iwamoto T, Nakajima C, Nishiuchi Y, et al. Genetic diversity of *Mycobacterium avium* subsp *hominissuis* strains isolated from humans, pigs, and human living environment. Infect Genet Evol 2011. [Epub ahead of print.]
36. Tortoli E, Brunello F, Cagni AE, et al. *Mycobacterium genavense* in AIDS patients, report of 24 cases in Italy and review of the literature. Eur J Epidemiol 1998;14:219–24.
37. Doggett JS, Strasfeld L. Disseminated Mycobacterium genavense with pulmonary nodules in a kidney transplant recipient: case report and review of the literature. Transpl Infect Dis 2011;13:38–43.
38. Miyoshi H, Tamura G, Satoh T, Disseminated Mycobacterium genavense infection in a healthy boy. Hum Pathol 2010;41:1646–9.
39. Napier JE, Hinrichs SH, Lampen F, et al. An outbreak of avian mycobacteriosis caused by *Mycobacterium intracellulare* in little blue penguins (*Eudyptula minor*). J Zoo Wildl Med 2009;40:680–6.
40. Kik MJ, Houwers DJ, Dinkla A. *Mycobacterium intermedium* granulomatous pneumonia in a green oropendola (Psarocolius viridis). Vet Rec 2010;167:219–20.
41. Gaukler SM, Linz GM, Sherwood JS, et al. *Escherichia coli*, *Salmonella*, and *Mycobacterium avium* subsp *paratuberculosis* in wild European starlings at a Kansas cattle feedlot. Avian Dis 2009;53:544–51.
42. Travis EK, Junge RE, Terrell SP. Infection with *Mycobacterium simiae* complex in four captive Micronesian kingfishers. J Am Vet Med Assoc 2007;230:1524–9.
43. Vitali SD, Eden PA, Payne KL, et al. An outbreak of mycobacteriosis in Gouldian finches caused by *Mycobacterium peregrinum*. Vet Clin North Am Exot Anim Pract 2006;9:519–22.
44. Carpenter JW. Exotic animal formulary. St Louis (MO): Elsevier Saunders; 2005.
45. Foldenauer U, Curd S, Zulauf I, et al. Ante mortem diagnosis of mycobacterial infection by liver biopsy in a budgerigar (*Melopsittacus undulatus*). Schweizer Archiv für Tierheilkunde 2007;149:273–6.
46. Sharma SJ, Mohan A. Multidrug-resistant tuberculosis. Indian J Med Res 2004;120:354–76.
47. Griffith DE. Therapy of non-tuberculous mycobacterial disease. Curr Opin Infect Dis 2007;20:198–203.
48. Esteban J, Ortiz-Pérez A. Current treatment of atypical mycobacteriosis. Exp Opin Pharm 2009;10:2787–99.

49. Carpenter JW, Olsen JH, Randle-Port M, et al. Pharmacokinetics of azithromycin in the blue and gold macaw (*Ara ararauna*) after intravenous and oral administration. J Zoo Wildl Med 2005;36:606–9.

50. Flammer K, Aucoin DP, Whitt DA. Intramuscular and oral disposition of enrofloxacin in African grey parrots following single and multiple doses. J Vet Pharmacol Ther 1991;14:359–66.

51. Nuermberger E, Grosset J. Pharmacokinetic and pharmacodynamic issues in the treatment of mycobacterial infections. Eur J Clin Microb Infect Dis 2004;23:243–55.

52. Katoch VM. Infections due to non-tuberculous mycobacteria (NTM). Indian J Med Res 2004;120:290–304.

53. Tomioka H. Present status and future prospects of chemotherapeutics for intractable infections due to *Mycobacterium avium* complex. Curr Drug Discov Technol 2004;1: 255–68.

54. Bammann RH, Zamarioli LA, Pinto VS, et al. High prevalence of drug-resistant tuberculosis and other mycobacteria among HIV-infected patients in Brazil: a systematic review. Mem Inst Oswaldo Cruz 2010;105:838–41.

55. Doucet-Populaire F, Buriánková K, Weiser J, Pernodet JL. Natural and acquired macrolide resistance in mycobacteria. Curr Drug Targets Infect Disord 2002;2:355–70.

56. Scholan EM, Pratt WB. The antimicrobial drugs. New York: Oxford University Press; 2000.

57. Sarkar S, Suresh MR. An overview of tuberculosis chemotherapy: a literature review. J Pharm Pharm Sci 2011;14:148–61.

58. Alcaide F, Pfyffer GE, Telenti A. Role of embB in natural and acquired resistance to Ethambutol in mycobacteria. Antimicrob Agent Chemother 1997;41:2270–3.

59. Baghdadi JE, Orlova M, Alter A, et al. An autosomal dominant major gene confers predisposition to pulmonary tuberculosis in adults. J Exp Med 2006;203:1679–84.

60. Chavez F, Alonso-Sanz M, Rebollo MJ, et al. rpoB mutations as an epidemiologic marker in rifampin-resistant mycobacterium tuberculosis. Int J Tuberc Lung Dis 2000;4:765–70.

61. Almeida Da Silva PE, Palomino JC. Molecular basis and mechanisms of drug resistance in *Mycobacterium tuberculosis*: classical and new drugs. J Antimicrob Chemother 2011;66:1417–30.

62. Inagaki T, Yagi T, Ichikawa K, et al. Evaluation of a rapid detection method of clarithromycin resistance genes in Mycobacterium avium complex isolates. Antimicrob Chemother 2011;66:722–9.

63. Ramaswamy SV, Amin AG, Goksel S. Molecular genetic analysis of nucleotide polymorphisms associated with ethambutol resistance in human isolates of *Mycobacterium tuberculosis*. Antimicrob Agents Chemother 2000;44:326–36.

Diagnosis of Mycobacterial Infections in the Exotic Pet Patient with Emphasis on Birds

Bob Dahlhausen, DVM, MS[a],*, Diego Soler Tovar, DVM, MS[b],
Miguel D. Saggese, DVM, MS, PhD[c]

KEYWORDS

- *Mycobacterium* • Diagnosis • Serology • Imaging
- Polymerase chain reaction • Culture • Birds • Reptiles
- Amphibians • Fish

The term "mycobacteriosis" encompasses a variety of infectious diseases of animals caused by bacteria of the genus *Mycobacterium*. Mycobacteriosis is a chronic, debilitating disease and usually of systemic presentation. More than 35 species in the genus *Mycobacterium* can cause mycobacteriosis in exotic pets (see article by Mark D. Schrenzel elsewhere in this issue for further exploration of this topic). The wide range of possible clinical signs and physical exam findings in the exotic pet with mycobacteriosis can make the antemortem diagnosis inconsistent and challenging. Proper sample collection and test modality in relation to the state of the disease process are essential in confirming a diagnosis of mycobacteriosis (see article by Mark D. Schrenzel elsewhere in this issue for further exploration of this topic).[1-5] Ultimately, clinicians can determine a presumptive diagnosis of mycobacteriosis based on history, clinical signs, imaging, hematology, serology, and other complementary ancillary tests. However, the definitive etiologic diagnosis of mycobacteriosis relies on the correct identification of the mycobacteria through its investigation by microbiological and molecular diagnostic methods. In this article, the clinical and etiologic diagnoses of mycobacteriosis in exotic pets are reviewed. As most data come from case reports and research conducted on birds, this group constitutes the

B.D. is owner-operator of Veterinary Molecular Diagnostics, Inc.
The authors have nothing to disclose.
[a] Veterinary Molecular Diagnostic, Inc, 5989 Meijer Drive, Suite 5, Milford, OH 45150, USA
[b] College of Agricultural Sciences, Universidad de La Salle, Bogotá, Colombia
[c] College of Veterinary Medicine, Western University of Health Sciences, 309 East Second Street, Pomona, CA 91766, USA
* Corresponding author.
E-mail address: drbob@one.net

Vet Clin Exot Anim 15 (2012) 71–83
doi:10.1016/j.cvex.2011.11.003
1094-9194/12/$ – see front matter © 2012 Published by Elsevier Inc.

main emphasis of our review. However, the diagnostic principles and techniques discussed here can be applied to other nonavian exotic pet patients.

CLINICAL SIGNS OF MYCOBACTERIOSIS

Mycobacteria can enter the organism through the oral, respiratory, and dermal routes. Infections initiated via ingestion of the organism can invade the intestinal tract, causing an eventual bacteremia and hematogeneous spread to the liver and other organs. Inhalation of the organism may produce lesions mainly in the lungs and air sacs, but subsequent dissemination through serosal surfaces to other organs may also occur. Less commonly, local skin infections manifest as discrete cutaneous lesions, especially in reptiles and fish.[6-8] In these species, mycobacteria are thought to be contracted through defects in the integument.[6-8] The clinical signs of myco-bacterial diseases are often subtle until late in the course of the disease and are not pathognomonic of mycobacteriosis. In most cases, a consistent and accurate diagnosis early in the course of the disease is difficult. Mycobacteriosis should be considered in the differential diagnosis of any exotic pet with chronic disease characterized by weight loss, an inflammatory leukogram, and organ enlarge-ment.[6-15] Chronic emaciation, muscle wasting, loss of subcutaneous and intracoe-lomic fat, poor-quality integument and skin appendages, diarrhea, dyspnea, biliver-dinuria, seizures, and paralysis are nonspecific but often observed findings in exotic pets with mycobacteriosis.[6-15] Subcutaneous granulomas, organomegaly, a pro-found leukocytosis, and the cytologic presence of acid-fast bacteria are strong indicators of the disease.[6-15] Mycobacteriosis should also be considered in those patients with dermatologic lesions such as masses and ulcers and with enlargement of joints, especially for those with negative results for fungal and aerobic/anaerobic bacteriologic cultures. Mycobacteriosis should also be suspected in cases of acute deaths.[9,16-18] However, sudden death is a rare occurrence and most likely represents a result of an undiagnosed chronic presentation or undetected clinical signs by the owner. Death might occur after an unrecognized, insidious disease course usually taking several weeks to months. Mycobacteriosis is rarely the cause of death in exotic pets without signs of chronic, consumptive disease.

In piscine and amphibian species, aquatic mycobacteria can cause variable clinical signs similar to diseases caused by other infectious, parasitic, and metabolic etiologies and can also manifest as acute or chronic disease.[6-8,10] Affected fish and amphibians may also exhibit an altered balance, swimming or floating separated from other individuals in the tank, decreased productivity, and dermatologic lesions such as missing scales and/or abnormal pigmentation of the skin.[6-8,10] Nodular skin lesions may be present, which often ulcerate or bleed. Additionally, there may be individuals with exophthalmia, abdominal distention, and skeletal deformities (such as spinal curvatures) as result of the chronic inflammatory process of these organs and surrounding anatomic structures.[7,8]

Readers are referred to other articles in this issue by Reavill and Schmidt, Mark A. Mitchell, Heatley and Martinho, and Diane E. McClure for further exploration of this topic.

GROSS PATHOLOGY FINDINGS

Postmortem examination of any exotic pet should be pursued following a systematic examination of the whole body. Adequate representative tissue samples should be taken during necropsy and gross pathology investigation for cytology, microbiology, histopathology, toxicology, and molecular diagnosis. Cross nucleic acid contamination is not prevented by sterilization alone. DNA can remain on the instruments and cause false-positive polymerase chain reaction results if highly sensitive molecular diagnosis and molecular characterization is pursued. Prevention of cross nucleic acid contamination can be prevented by using new sets of disposable instruments or by previous treatment with formalin and bleach to degrade nucleic acids.

A diagnosis of mycobacteriosis is strongly supported on histopathology results demonstrating the presence of typical lesions and acid-fast organisms by Ziehl-Neelsen staining. However, the correct identification of the species and strain of mycobacteria should be pursued by culture and DNA probes with nucleic acid amplification. The location of the primary lesion is a possible indicator of the route of exposure. Intestinal lesions suggests an oral route of infection through contaminated food or water. Lesions in the lungs and other areas of the respiratory tract suggest inhalation as the route of exposure.[19] In disseminated mycobacteriosis the primary lesion may not always be clearly identified.[20]

Gross pathology findings in birds usually include emaciation, absence of subcutaneous and mesenteric fat, and severe atrophy of the pectoral muscles.[21] Hepatomegaly and splenomegaly are also frequent findings. A classic presentation includes the observation of white or yellowish nodules in the lungs, spleen, intestine, air sac, bone marrow, and, more rarely, the heart, gonads, central nervous system (CNS), skin, and joints.[4,9,20–23] Affected birds may not always evidence this classic presentation. The diagnosis of mycobacteriosis may be misled if based only upon the presence of these classic lesions. Lepromatous or diffuse granulomatous inflammation of the liver and spleen may manifest as diffuse enlargement and discoloration of the organ without evident foci of caseous necrosis.[23]

In reptiles, grayish or whitish nodules can usually be seen in several organs (digestive, respiratory, and genitourinary tracts; heart; spleen; peritoneal surface; and CNS) and in the subcutaneous space.[12,13,24,25] Unlike mammals, calcified lesions are not observed in reptiles, amphibians, and birds but have been described in fish.[7,8,12,13,21,24,25]

Lesions of mycobacteriosis in fish are commonly found along the intestinal wall and skin, showing grayish-white miliary granulomas of varying consistency; however the spleen, kidneys, liver, heart, and gonads may also be affected. Edema and peritonitis may be present. In severe cases, the visceral organs are enlarged and fused by the presence of whitish membranes around the mesentery.[7,8]

Amyloid deposits are sometimes observed in parenchymatous organs (liver, kidney, and spleen) from exotic pet birds affected with mycobacteriosis.[20,21,23] This can easily be identified by Congo Red staining. Under polarized light, amyloid fibrils can be seen as green birefringence in a dark background. Amyloidoisis is a pathologic condition that results after chronic inflammatory processes but is not pathognomonic of mycobacteriosis. A full review of gross and microscopic pathology is beyond the scope of this article and the topic is thoroughly reviewed in other sections of this special issue on mycobacteriosis and references therein.

Readers are referred to other articles in this issue by Reavill and Schmidt, Shivaprasad and Palmieri, Diane E. McClure, and Mark A. Mitchell for further exploration of this topic.

HEMATOLOGY AND CLINICAL BIOCHEMISTRY

Hematologic changes in exotic pets affected by mycobacteriosis usually reflect the chronic inflammatory condition of the disease. These changes in birds are often not evident until the disease is well advanced.[5,11,26] When present, severe changes in the hemogram often indicate the end stage of the disease process.[5,18] The packed cell volume is often decreased, reflecting an anemia of chronic disease. Corresponding polychromasia, hypochromasia, and anisocytosis are usually present. An increase in packed cell volume may however be observed in cases of primary respiratory mycobacteriosis.[27] Although abnormalities of the hemogram may be few and variable, disseminated mycobacteriosis typically produces a moderate-to-marked increase in the white blood cell count. A persistent leukocytosis is characterized by neutrophilia/heterophilia and monocytosis.[4,5,9,11,26] A reactive lymphocytosis may also be present. Exotic pets with localized lesions in the skin may not show detectable changes in the hemogram. Alterations in the serum chemistry panel are variable and often unremarkable. In birds, hepatic mycobacteriosis may produce increases in enzyme activities such as alanine aminotransferase, aspartate aminotransferase, and lactate dehydrogenase.[5,9,11,28] Although liver enzymes may be mildly to moderately elevated, they can be normal in the face of severe hepatic disease.[5,27,28] These enzymes are also present in a variety of other tissues such as muscle, kidney, and heart. Plasma protein electrophoresis results are also inconsistent.[29] A polyclonal gammaglobulinopathy may be present early in the disease process in birds and reptiles.[30–34] Hyperglobulinemia, hyperproteinemia, and elevated blood fibrinogen may be present. When abnormal, blood albumin levels are usually decreased. These hematologic abnormalities, however, can be present in many other inflammatory and chronic disease conditions.[30,31,33,34] The main value of clinical biochemistry and plasma protein electrophoresis is to detect and monitor the course of chronic inflammatory disease, but by themselves they are not useful for the etiologic diagnosis of mycobacterial infections.

HUMORAL ASSAYS

Serologic techniques provide a less invasive method for the diagnosis of mycobacteriosis. The need for species-specific antigens and effectiveness in detecting only late-stage infections has limited their broad application to many exotic species. Serologic assays such as hemagglutination (HA), complement fixation, enzyme-linked immunosorbent assay (ELISA), and Western blot analysis have been used to variably identify infected birds.[35–40] Mechanisms that allow mycobacteria to evade the host immune system make application of humoral response assays most useful in late-stage infections. The need for specialized antigens targeted to individual species and the broad spectrum of mycobacteria involved in cases of mycobacteriosis in exotic pets limit the broad application of these methods. Furthermore, these tests are not commercially available. The greater applicability of in-house developed serologic techniques could be as an initial screening tool for *Mycobacterium* exposure in large captive populations of a single species. To the best of the author's knowledge, no humoral assays have been developed for reptiles and amphibians, although monoclonal antibodies have been developed for 2 species of fish with mycobacteriosis.[41] HA is a rapid assay that can test whole blood or serum. It has been used for diagnosing infections in waterfowl, poultry, raptors, and cranes.[1,26] HA tests are, however, highly species specific. Specialized antigens are required for reliable results. Complement fixation titers (≥1:20) have also been used to confirm exposure and infection by *Mycobacterium avium* in grey-cheeked parakeets (*Brotogeris pyrrhopterus*) and doves (Columbidae).[39,42] ELISAs have been useful in detecting mycobacterial infections in avian species. Sensitive and specific ELISAs exist for infection in waterfowl.[1,38] While ELISAs have been developed for testing specific avian populations, they have not been effective early in the disease process. Furthermore, antibody production may cease or decrease in advanced stages of infection.[38,39] An ELISA recently developed for waterfowl showed a low sensitivity

(76.9%) and specificity (55.6%) for the diagnosis of mycobacteriosis.[38] Broad application of humoral assays is limited by the need for highly species-specific antigens, the wide range of species of mycobacteria involved in mycobacteriosis, and the diversity of exotic pets. Western blot analysis has been used to assess the humoral response of ring-neck doves (*Streptopelia risoria*) exposed to *M avium* subsp *avium*.[40] A sensitivity of 88.24% and a specificity of 100% were achieved using this method. The findings of this study indicate that Western blot analysis can be a useful screening tool for the antemortem identification of infected birds.

CELLULAR-BASED ASSAYS

Intradermal tuberculin tests have been used to reliably diagnosis mycobacteriosis in domestic poultry.[11] A small volume (0.1 mL) of avian purified protein derivative tuberculin is injected into the wattle or comb and assessed 48 to 72 hours later. This method however is unreliable in a number of avian species including pigeons, geese, quail, and raptors.[2,11,43] Intradermal skin testing in these species is frequently associated with false negatives, especially in the early and late stages of the disease process. Results of intradermal tuberculosis testing also correlate poorly with the presence of disease in psittacine species and other exotic pets.

RADIOLOGY AND OTHER IMAGING TECHNIQUES

The diverse nature of mycobacterial infections in exotic pets makes radiology an inconsistent diagnostic tool, especially in the early stages of disease.[3,14] Radiographic evaluation may, however, help substantiate a presumptive diagnosis of mycobacteriosis.[3,13,14,44] Observed radiographic changes can include coelomic and organ enlargement, pulmonary granulomas, and lytic bone lesions. Hepatosplenomegaly and gaseous dilation of intestinal loops is often observed in affected species with gastrointestinal mycobacteriosis. Gastrointestinal contrast studies may demonstrate a thickened and irregular wall of the small intestine. Granulomas may be identified within the coelom, lungs, or bones. A nodular granulomatous pericarditis and myocarditis causing severe hydropericardium and cardiac tamponade were evident in infected Gang Gang cockatoos (*Callocephalon fimbriatum*).[45] Given that granulomas do not mineralize in birds and reptiles, it may be difficult to distinguish lesions caused by mycobacteria from similar soft tissue densities such as those produced by aspergillosis and neoplasia.[11] In birds, radiographic findings involving bone include lysis and/or sclerosis consistent with osteomyelitis, osteophytosis around arthritic joints, pathologic fractures, and increased opacity in endosteal bone density. Anatomic regions most commonly affected are the midshaft region of long bones including the humerus, tibia, ulna, and, infrequently, femur. An unusual report of chondritis, osteitis, and osteomyelitis was described in the nasal bone of a wood duck (*Aix sponsa*) with mycobacteriosis.[46] Ultrasonography and alternate imaging methods, such as computed tomography, are also potentially useful diagnostics for identifying these associated changes. Ultrasonography reveals abnormalities in the size and architecture of the liver and spleen and facilitates fine needle biopsy. Magnetic resonance imaging is a useful diagnostic procedure to detect brain lesions in animals with progressive neurologic signs attributed to mycobacteriosis.[11]

ENDOSCOPY AND BIOPSY

Endoscopy allows direct visualization of infiltrative lesions in the abdominal or coelomic cavity and respiratory tract. Coelomic endoscopic examination is a useful technique for identifying lesions on the serosal surface of the liver, spleen, intestine, lung, and air sacs. Granulomas may be visualized as white, yellow, or tan round masses, which are soft and easily biopsied. Enlargement of the liver, kidneys, and spleen is also a common finding during coelomic and abdominal endoscopic examination of exotic pets with mycobacteriosis. Samples of abnormal tissues or granulomas can be investigated to confirm the diagnosis of mycobacteriosis. Additionally, it allows the sampling of lesions for cytologic or histopathologic examination, acid-resistant staining, culture, and molecular tests.[4,5,9,11] Histopathologic examination, culture, or PCR are preferred methods for confirming the presence of the organism in these samples, followed by molecular characterization. The liver is often considered a tissue of choice when diagnosing avian mycobacteriosis.[1,3,4] In a study of Japanese quail (*Coturnix japonica*) experimentally inoculated with M avium, results demonstrated that culture and PCR of liver, spleen, and intestinal tissue samples exhibited 100% correlation with infection.[47] Naturally infected ring-neck doves (*Streptopelia risoria*) had more splenic lesions containing acid-fast organisms than hepatic lesions, suggesting that splenic biopsy may have greater potential for the antemortem diagnosis of mycobacterial infection in this species.[5,20] The same study demonstrated that liver biopsy alone cannot be used to rule out mycobacteriosis.[5] Sensitivity was also higher for postmortem examination of multiple liver sections than of a single biopsy section. Obtaining multiple biopsy sections from liver and other affected organs may increase mycobacterial detection in the exotic patient with systemic mycobacteriosis.[5]

CYTOLOGY

Microscopic examination of cytologic samples from target organs, skin, and fecal matter is useful as results are immediately available and, if positive, provide a presumptive diagnosis of mycobacterial infection. Conversely, this screening tool does not take the place of culture, histopathology, or DNA probes for defining the diagnosis.[48] Giemsa-stained preparations may reveal macrophages with intracellular, negative-staining "ghost" cells representing unstained mycobacteria in the cytoplasm. Acid-fast stains such as Ziehl-Neelsen (Z-N) are commonly used to identify mycobacterial organisms. They appear as pink-red rods, beaded rods to almost coccoid in nature.[48] The Truant (Truant AFB stain kit, Fisher Scientific Inc., Pittsburgh, PA, USA) (Auramine O-Rhodamine B) fluorochromic stain, however, appears superior to Z-N for identifying the organism in cytologic as well as histopathologic samples. Truant-stained tissue samples of infected quail compared more favorably with positive culture results than did standard Z-N–stained samples (95.7% and 82.6%, respectively).[49] Unlike mammalian infections, granulomatous lesions in avian species typically contain large numbers of acid-fast–laden macrophages and intralesional organisms (see article by Shivaprasad and Palmieri elsewhere in this issue for further exploration of this topic).[11,21] A minimum of approximately 10,000 organisms/mL is required for detection by these methods.[15] Mycobacterial infections in psittacine birds commonly involve the gastrointestinal tract (see article by Shivaprasad and Palmieri elsewhere in this issue for further exploration of this topic).[11,21] Granulomas often communicate with the intestinal lumen, allowing the organism to be shed in the feces. Microscopic examination of stained fecal smears may aid the diagnosis by revealing acid-fast mycobacteria. Low sensitivity is a disadvantage. Fecal shedding of the organism is inconsistent and tends to occur in the latter stages of the disease.[47,49] A negative smear therefor does not rule out infection. Examination of Z-N–stained intestinal aspirates from infected ring-neck doves (*Streptopelia risoria*) failed to detect infection in most birds.[20] In infected Japanese quail, fecal stain sensitivities were 7.2% for Z-N– and 30.4% for Truant-stained samples compared to fecal culture.[47,49] The identification of mycobacteria in fecal samples can be optimized by repeated fecal culture and Truant acid-fast staining.[47,49] Fluorochrome staining such as Truant stain is highly sensitive (sensitivity and specificity for tissue samples of 95.7% and 100% and for fecal samples of 30.4% and 98.4%, respectively).[2,47,49] Care must also be taken in interpreting positive fecal smears. The acid-fast stain is not a specific test. Nonpathogenic mycobacteria, which can be transient gastrointestinal inhabitants or environmental contaminants, may be identified.[15] Positive acid-fast cytology should be confirmed by culture or DNA probe analysis. Cytologic examination of sputum or tracheal and lung washes/exudates may reveal the presence of acid-fast bacilli in exotic pets with respiratory mycobacteriosis.

CULTURE

The genus *Mycobacterium* includes more than 150 species.[50] They all belong to the family Mycobacteriacea.[51] Historically, mycobacterial culture of tissue specimens has been the gold standard for a confirmed diagnosis of infection.[51] The slow growth of the mycobacterial organism is the greatest obstacle to rapidly confirming a diagnosis. Culture of mycobacteria is not always successful and is time-consuming to complete.[51] A minimum incubation period of 1 to 4 and up to 8 weeks is required for visible colonies to appear. Some strains of *M avium* complex (MAC) may take as long as 6 months before becoming identifiable. On the contrary, some rapid growing mycobacteria, such as *M abscessus, M fortuitum,* and *M chelonae,* may yield positive results in less than 1 week.[51] The development of radiometric culture systems allows for faster and increased recovery of the mycobacterial organism. This is especially useful for isolation of *M genavense*. The organism is a common pathogen of pet birds that shows very slow and inconsistent growth and is difficult to isolate by standard culture techniques.[52–55] In one study, only 3 of 34 *M genavense* isolates grew on conventional media, while radiometric culture supported the growth of 23 of 34 isolates.[54] *M avium* subsp *avium* is more readily cultured in broth and other liquid and solid media as well. The presence of an adequate number of microorganisms is essential for obtaining a positive culture. A concentration greater than 10 viable organisms/mL is required for a positive culture.[15] In cases with an uneven or localized distribution of microorganisms in the parenchyma of affected organs, a false negative result may occur if the selected section of tissue does not contain a sufficient number of microorganisms. Fecal culture may confirm infection in the individual bird but does have practical limitations. *Mycobacterium* is generally shed only in the latter stages of the disease and, when it does occur, is intermittent in nature. Mycobacteria were isolated from 53% (69 of 130) of fecal samples from birds in a controlled inoculation study.[47,49] Fecal culture was positive more often late in the course of the study, indicating that the culture-positive rate was higher later in the course of the infection.[47,49] Careful fecal sample collection is also necessary to prevent contamination from environmental organisms. Although the specificity of fecal culture is generally high, the sensitivity of this method is low.[2,9,11] Before attempting a culture for the isolation of mycobacteria, samples must be decontaminated to prevent the growth of other bacteria.[51] Selective decontamination can be easily achieved with NaOH, sodium dodecyl sulfate, N-acetyl-L-cysteine, sodium hydroxide, oxalic acid, trisodium phosphate zefirano, sulfuric acid, and chloride hexadecylpyridinium.[2,51,56] Mycobacterial cultures in solid medium can be easily indentified. Colonies usually are cream colored, but some may produce a pigment, depending on the species of mycobacteria involved and the culture medium used.[51,56]

Commonly used culture media for mycobacteria include Lowenstein-Jensen, modified Herrold egg yolk medium, Stonebrink, Petragnani, and liquid media such as Middlebrook 7H11, Middlebrook 7H10, and Middlebrook 7H9.[48,51,56] The addition of mycobactin, sheep blood, and charcoal to acidified agar media has been found to promote the growth of *M genavense* in solid medium.[57] A combination of different culture media and culturing conditions increases the likelihood of positive isolates.[2,11,15]

Further characterization of isolates relies on biochemical tests, serum agglutination, and molecular methodologies. Biochemical tests, including pigment production, growth on MacConkey agar (without crystal violet), sodium chloride tolerance of 5% nitrate reduction, growth on thiophene hydrazoic acid-2-carboxylic acid, pyrazinamide deamination, urease production, niacin production, hydrolysis of Tween 80 (Fisher Scientific Inc., Pittsburgh, PA, USA), inhibition of glycerol, iron intake, arylsulfatase, catalase production, and the time and temperature required for optimum growth, contribute to characterizing the species and strain characteristics involved.[51,56] Molecular methods are, however, rapidly replacing these microbiological techniques for a confirmed diagnosis.

POLYMERASE CHAIN REACTION

Improvements in nucleic acid detection methodology, like DNA probes, PCR, and PCR-restriction fragment length polymorphism have revolutionized the speed and quality of detection of mycobacterial organisms in clinical samples.[58,59] Molecular methods have demonstrated high sensitivity and specificity for confirmatory mycobacterial testing. PCR can detect very low numbers of viable or nonviable organisms, distinguish individual mycobacterial species, and determine drug resistance patterns of the organism.[47,49] Restriction fragment length polymorphism analysis and multiplex PCR methods can discriminate between intraspecies genotypes, which is particularly useful for epidemiologic studies (see article by Mark D. Schrenzel elsewhere in this issue for further exploration of this topic).[50,60,61] PCR is rapid, specific, and inexpensive. It can be performed on any tissue including biopsy or necropsy tissue samples, fecal or cloacal swabs, and formalin-fixed paraffin-embedded sections. Conclusive results can be obtained rapidly within days compared with culture, which may require weeks to months to complete. These technologies are an excellent diagnostic alternative to more conventional methods. PCR has become the preferred method of antemortem and postmortem diagnosis of *Mycobacterium* in clinical samples. In the past, most cases of avian infection were assumed to be caused by the MAC (see article by Shivaprasad and Palmieri elsewhere in this issue for further exploration of this topic).[15,54] Molecular techniques have identified the role of fastidious mycobacteria, primarily *M genavense*, in avian species. *M genavense* is responsible for the majority of pet bird infections (in parrots and songbirds up to 80%), while MAC accounts for only 5% to 20% (see article by Shivaprasad and Palmieri elsewhere in this issue for further exploration of this topic).[15,54] Molecular methods are replacing culture as the gold standard diagnostic test for *Mycobacterium* spp, especially those organisms whose genomic sequences have been documented (GenBank database). In a study of Japanese quail (*Coturnix japonica*) experimentally inoculated with *M avium*, results demonstrated that culture and PCR of target tissue samples (liver, spleen, and intestine) were 96% and 100% sensitive in identifying the infection, respectively.[3] Commercial nucleic acid hybridization probes have become the method of choice for distinction between *M avium* (and its different subspecies), *M intracellulare,* and *M genavense.*[62–67] The sensitivity, specificity, and reproducibility of PCR assays are influenced by the quality and quantity of DNA in the test sample. Fecal samples and cloacal swabs may contain enzymes that degrade sample DNA and inhibitors that interfere with the PCR. Inhibitory agents particularly prevalent in the fecal samples

Table 1 Diagnostic laboratories that offer testing of avian samples for *Mycobacterium* sp	
Test	Laboratory
PCR	Veterinary Molecular Diagnostics 1-513-576-1808 Submit feces, vent swab, suspect target tissue/s
PCR	Washington State University Animal Disease Diagnostic Laboratory 1-509-335-9696 Submit feces, suspect target tissue/s
Culture	National Jewish Medical and Research Center, Denver, CO Culture and sensitivity testing 1-303-398-1339; www.rjc.org Contact laboratory for submission instructions

Data from Lennox AM. Mycobacteriosis in companion psittacine birds: a review. J Avian Med Surg 2007;21:181–7.

include hemoglobin, bile acids, proteins, and complex polysaccharides originating from dietary material. To reduce this interference, DNA extraction protocols with heat or detergent cationic surfactants C_{18}-carboxypropylbetaine are recommended.[47,49] The use of enzymatic lysis alone or combined with thermal disruption of the mycobacterial wall through high temperatures, successive cycles of freezing and boiling, and the use of mechanical membrane disruption with zirconia beads increases the yield of nucleic acids.[47,49]

In the controlled infectivity study of Japanese quail, PCR was inadequate for the detection of *M avium* in fecal samples. While the specificity of PCR compared with fecal culture was greater than 95%, sensitivity was only 20.3%. Refinements in DNA extraction techniques and PCR procedures have enhanced the clinical utility of this method for antemortem diagnosis of mycobacteriosis in birds and other exotic pets.Currently, most species of mycobacterium affecting exotic pets can be identified by PCR and sequencing of species specific genes or insertion sequences.[62–67] Molecular epidemiology studies can also be conducted from archival mycobacteriosis cases in pathologic collections.[67,68]

SUMMARY

Clinicians can make a presumptive diagnosis of mycobacteriosis in exotic pets based on history, clinical signs, imaging, hematology, serology, and other complementary ancillary tests. Histopathology can be useful to confirm the presence of acid fast microorganisms in granulomatous and/or lepromatous lesions typical of mycobacterial infections. However, the definitive etiologic diagnosis of mycobacteriosis relies on the correct identification of the mycobacteria involved by classic microbiologic and, more recently, molecular diagnostic methods. Mycobacterial culture or PCR analyses are the most sensitive and specific laboratory tests for a definitive diagnosis. Examination of multiple tissues and the use of several different diagnostic techniques significantly increase the probability of diagnosis of mycobacteriosis. Diagnostic laboratories that offer testing of avian samples for *Mycobacterium* in avian samples are listed in **Table 1**.

REFERENCES

1. Cromie RL, Brown MA, Forbes N, et al. A comparison and evaluation of techniques for diagnosis of avian tuberculosis in wildfowl. Avian Pathol 1993;22:617–30.

2. Aranaz A, Liebana E, Mateos A, et al. Laboratory diagnosis of avian mycobacteriosis. Sem Avian Exot Pet Med 1997;6:9–17.

3. Tell L, Foley J, Needham M, et al. Diagnosis of avian mycobacteriosis: comparison of culture, acid-fast stains, and polymerase chain reaction for the identification of *Mycobacterium avium* in experimentally inoculated Japanese quail (*Coturnix coturnix japonica*). Avian Dis 2003;47:444–52.

4. Lennox AM. Mycobacteriosis in companion psittacine birds: a review. J Avian Med Surg 2007;21:181–7.

5. Saggese MD, Tizard I, Phalen DN. Comparison of sampling methods, culture, acid-fast stain, and polymerase chain reaction assay for the diagnosis of mycobacteriosis in ring-neck doves (*Streptopelia risoria*). J Avian Med Surg 2010;24:263–71.

6. Noga EJ. Fish diseases: diagnosis and treatment. Ames (IO): Blackwell; 2010.

7. Gauthier DT, Rhodes MW. Mycobacteriosis in fishes: a review. Vet J 2009;180: 33–47.

8. Jacobs J, Stine C, Baya A, et al. A review of mycobacteriosis in marine fish. J Fish Dis 2009;32:119–30.

9. Van der Heyden N. Clinical manifestations of mycobacteriosis in pet birds. Sem Avian Exot Pet Med 1997;6:18–24.

10. Smith S. Mycobacterial Infections in Pet Fish. Sem Avian Exot Pet Med 1997;6:40–5.

11. Tell LA, Woods L, Cromie RL. Mycobacteriosis in birds. Rev Sci Tech 2001;20:180–203.

12. Soldati G, Lu Z, Vaughan L, et al. Detection of Mycobacteria and Chlamydia in granulomatous inflammation of reptiles: a retrospective study. Vet Pathol 2004;41:388–97.

13. Rosenthal KL, Mader DR. Bacterial diseases. In: Mader DR, editor. Reptile medicine and surgery. St Louis: Elsevier; 2006. p. 227–38.

14. Pollock CG. Implications of mycobacteria in clinical disorders. In: Harrison GJ, Lightfoot TL, editors. Clinical avian medicine. Tampa (FL): Florida Spix; 2006. p. 681–8.

15. Converse K. Avian tuberculosis. In: Thomas NJ, Hunter DB, Atkinson CT, editors. Infectious diseases of wild birds. Oxford (UK): Blackwell; 2007. p. 125–9.

16. Kock N, Kock R, Wambua J, et al. *Mycobacterium avium*-related epizootic in free-ranging lesser flamingos in Kenya. J Wildl Dis 1999;35:297–300.

17. Silveira L, Fowler M. Order Anseriformes (ducks, geese, swans): bacterial diseases. In: Fowler M, Cubas Z, editors. Biology, medicine, and surgery of South American wild animals. Aimes (IO): Iowa State University Press; 2001. p. 91.

18. Riggs GL. White-winged wood duck (*Cairina scutulata*) species survival plan update. In: Proceedings of American Association of Zoo Veterinarians Annual Conference. Los Angeles (CA), 2008.

19. Soler D, Brieva C, Ribón W. Mycobacteriosis in wild birds: the potential risk disseminating a little-known infectious disease. Rev Salud Púb 2009;11:134–44.

20. Saggese MD, Riggs G, Tizard I, et al. Gross and microscopic findings and investigation of the aetiopathogenesis of mycobacteriosis in a captive population of white-winged ducks (*Cairina scutulata*). Avian Pathol 2007;36:415–22.

21. Schmidt RE, Reavill DR, Phalen DN. Pathology of pet and aviary birds. Ames (IO): Blackwell; 2003.

22. Gomez G, Saggese MD, Weeks BR, et al. Granulomatous encephalomyelitis and intestinal ganglionitis in a spectacled Amazon parrot (*Amazona albifrons*) infected with *Mycobacterium genavense*. J Comp Pathol 2011;144:219–22.

23. Saggese MD, Tizard I, Phalen DN. Mycobacteriosis in naturally infected ring-neck doves (*Streptopelia risoria*): investigation of the association between feather colour and susceptibility to infection, disease and lesions type. Avian Pathol 2008;37:443–50.

24. Agudelo A, Rodríguez G, Arias L. Identificación de *Mycobacterium* sp. en una población de tortugas morrocoy (*Geochelone carbonaria*) en cautiverio y en su entorno en un zoológico en la Sabana de Bogotá. Rev Med Vet 2008;15:21–38.
25. Jacobson ER. Infectious diseases and pathology of reptiles: color atlas and text. London: Taylor and Francis; 2007.
26. Hawkey C, Kock RA, Henderson GM. Hematological changes in domestic fowl (*Gallus gallus*) and cranes (Gruiformes) with *Mycobacterium avium* infection. Avian Pathol 1990;19:223–34.
27. Fudge AM. Avian complete blood count. In Fudge AM, editor. Laboratory medicine: avian and exotic pets. Philadelphia: WB Saunders; 2000. p. 90–8.
28. Janesch S. Diagnosis of avian hepatic disease. Semin Avian Exotic Pet Med 2000;9: 126–35.
29. Rosenthal K. Avian protein disorders. In: Fudge AM, editor. Laboratory medicine: avian and exotic pets. Philadelphia: WB Saunders; 2000. p. 171–3.
30. Tatum LM, Zaias J, Mealey BK, et al. Protein electrophoresis as a diagnostic and prognostic tool in raptor medicine. J Zoo Wildl Med 2000;31:497–502.
31. Zaias J, Cray C. Protein electrophoresis: a tool for the reptilian and amphibian practitioner. J Herp Med Surg 2004;12:30–2.
32. Cray C, Rodriguez M, Zaias J. Protein electrophoresis of psittacine plasma. Vet Clin Pathol 2007;36:64–72.
33. Gicking BS, Allen M, Kendal E. H, et al. Plasma protein electrophoresis of the Atlantic Loggerhead sea turtle (Caretta caretta). J Herpet Med Surg 2004;14:13–8.
34. Deem SL, Norton TM, Mitchell M, et al. Comparison of blood values in foraging, nesting, and stranded loggerhead turtles (*Caretta caretta*) along the coast of Georgia, USA. J Wildl Dis 2009;45:41–56.
35. Thoen CO. Tuberculosis. In: Calnek BW, editor. Diseases of poultry. 10th edition. Ames (IO): Iowa State University Press; 1997.
36. Cromie RL, Brown MJ, Forbes NA, et al. A comparison and evaluation of techniques for diagnosis of avian tuberculosis in wildfowl. Avian Pathol 1993;22:617–30.
37. Hoenerhoff M, Kiupel M, Sikarskie J, et al. Mycobacteriosis in an American Bald Eagle (Haliaeetus leucocephalus). Avian Dis 2004;48:437–41.
38. Zsivanovits H, Neumann U, Brown M, et al. Use of an enzyme-linked immunosorbent assay to diagnose avian tuberculosis in a captive collection of wildfowl. Avian Pathol 2004;33:571–5.
39. Phalen DN, Grimes JE, Phalen SW, et al. Serologic diagnosis of mycobacterial infections in birds (a preliminary report). Proc Assoc Avian Vet 1995;67–73.
40. Gray PL, Saggese MD, Phalen DN, et al. Humoral response to *Mycobacterium avium* subsp. *avium* in naturally infected ring-neck doves (*Streptopelia risoria*). Vet Immunol Immunopathol 2008;125:216–24.
41. Adams A, Thompson KD, McEwan H, et al. Development of monoclonal antibodies to *Mycobacterium* spp. isolated from Chevron snakehead and Siamese fighting fish. J Aqua Anim Health 1996;8:208–15.
42. Saggese MD, Phalen DN. Serological and histological findings in doves with mycobacteriosis. Proceedings of the 26th Association of Avian Veterinarians Conference. Monterrey (CA), 2005. p. 71–3.
43. Gerlach H. Bacteria. In: Ritchie B, Harrison G, Harrison L, editors. Avian medicine: principles and applications. Brentwood (TN): HBD Int; 1999. p. 949–83.
44. Silverman S. Diagnostic imaging. In: Mader DR, editor. Reptile medicine and surgery. St Louis: Elsevier; 2006.
45. Gelis S, Gill JH, Oldfield T. Mycobacteriosis in Gang Gang Cockatoos (*Callocephalon fimbriatum*). Vet Clin Exot Anim 2006;9:487–94.

46. Ferguson SH, Wallace LJ, Dunbar F. *Mycobacterium intracellulare (Battey bacillus)* infection in a Florida wood duck (*Aix sponsa*). Am Rev Respir Dis 1969;100:876–9.
47. Tell LA, Leutenegger CM, Larsen RS, et al. Real-time polymerase chain reaction testing for the detection of Mycobacterium genavense and Mycobacterium avium complex species in avian samples. Avian Dis 2003;47:1406–15.
48. Forbes BA, Sahm DF, Weissfeld AS. Mycobacteria. In Bailey and Scott's diagnostic microbiology. 10th edition. St Louis: Mosby; 1998. p. 715–50.
49. Tell LA, Foley J, Needham ML, et al. Comparison of four rapid DNA extraction techniques for conventional polymerase chain reaction testing of three *Mycobacterium* spp. that affect birds. Avian Dis 2003;47:1486–90.
50. Tortoli E. Impact of genotypic studies on mycobacterial taxonomy: the new mycobacteria of the 1990s. Clin Microbiol Rev 2003;16:319–54.
51. Mahon CR, Manuselis G, Lehman DC. Textbook of diagnostic microbiology. New York: Saunders; 2007.
52. Ramis A, Ferrer L, Aranaz A, et al. *Mycobacterium genavense* infection in canaries. Avian Dis 1996;40:246–51.
53. Buogo H, Bacciarini L, Robert N, et al. Presence of Mycobacterium genavense in birds. Schweiz Arch Tierheilkd 1997;139:397–402.
54. Hoop RK, Bottger EC, Pfyffer GE. Etiological agents of mycobacteriosis in pet birds between 1986 and 1995. J Clin Microbiol 1996;34:991–2.
55. Portaels F, Realini L, Bauwens I, et al. Mycobacteriosis caused by *Mycobacterium genavense* in birds kept in a zoo: 11-year survey. J Clin Microbiol 1996;34:319–23.
56. Brooks G, Butel J, Ornston L. Micobacterias. In: Jawetz E, Melnick J, Adelberg E, editors. Microbiología médica. 15th edition. México: Editorial Manual Moderno; 1996.
57. Realini L, De Ridder K, Hirschel B. Blood and charcoal added to acidified agar media promote the growth of *Mycobacterium genavense*. Diagn Microbiol Infect Dis 1999; 34:45–50.
58. Fries J, Patel R, Piessens W, et al. Genus- and species-specific DNA probes to identify mycobacteria using the polymerase chain reaction. Mol Cell Probes 1990;4:87–105.
59. Crawford, JT. Development of rapid techniques for identification of *M. avium* infections. Res Microbiol 1994;145:177–81.
60. Mazurek G, Hartman S, Zhang Y. Large DNA restriction fragment polymorphism in the *Mycobacterium avium M. intracellulare* complex: a potential epidemiologic tool. J Clin Microbiol 1993;31:390–4.
61. Devulder G, Pérouse de Montclos M, Flandrois JP. A multigene approach to phylogenetic analysis using the genus Mycobacterium as a model. Int J Syst Evol Microbiol 2005;55:293–302.
62. Kox LF, Jansen HM, Kuijper S, et al. Multiplex PCR assay for immediate identification of the infecting species in patients with mycobacterial disease. J Clin Microbiol 1997;35:1492–8.
63. Chevrier D, Oprisan G, Maresca A, et al. Isolation of a specific DNA fragment and development of a PCR-based method for the detection of *Mycobacterium genavense*. FEMS Immunol Med Microbiol 1999;23:243–52.
64. Shin SJ, Lee BS, Koh WJ, et al. Efficient differentiation of *Mycobacterium avium* complex species and subspecies by use of five-target multiplex PCR. J Clin Microbiol 2010;48:4057–62.
65. Gopinath K, Singh S. Multiplex PCR assay for simultaneous detection and differentiation of *Mycobacterium tuberculosis*, *Mycobacterium avium* complexes and other Mycobacterial species directly from clinical specimens. J Appl Microbiol 2009;107: 425–35.

66. Collins D, Cavaignac S, Lisle G. Use of four DNA insertion sequences to characterize strains of the *Mycobacterium avium* complex isolated from animals. Mol Cel Probes 1997;11:373–80.
67. Van Soolingen D, Bauer J, Ritacco V, et al. IS1245 restriction fragment length polymorphism typing of *Mycobacterium avium* isolates: proposal for standardization. J Clin Microbiol 1998;36:3051–4.
68. Pourahmad F, Thompson KD, Adams A, et al. Detection and identification of aquatic mycobacteria in formalin-fixed, paraffin-embedded fish tissues. J Fish Dis 2009;32: 409–19.

Mycobacteriosis in the Rabbit and Rodent

Diane E. McClure, DVM, PhD, DACLAM

KEYWORDS

- Mycobacteriosis • *Mycobacterium* • Tuberculosis
- Reservoir • Rabbit • Pygmy rabbit • Guinea pig • Rat
- Mice • Squirrel • Rodent

In general, mycobacteriosis causes few clinical concerns for pet rabbits and rodents. Overt mycobacteriosis is rarely reported in rodents and this chapter will review the few case reports of mycobacteriosis in rodents and rabbits. A brief review of rabbit and rodents used as animal models can provides insight to mycobacteriosis disease processes in these species. Finally, although rabbits and rodents are rarely clinically affected by mycobacteriosis, rabbits and rodents can serve as a potential reservoir between wildlife, domestic animals, and humans. The potential role of rabbits and rodents in the epidemiology of tuberculosis will be discussed.

SPONTANEOUS MYCOBACTERIOSIS—PYGMY RABBITS

The pygmy rabbit (*Brachylagus idahoensis*) (**Fig. 1**) is native to northeastern regions of the United States, southeastern Washington, southern Idaho, southwestern Montana, western Wyoming, western Utah, northern Nevada, northeastern California, and eastern Oregon (**Fig. 2**). A subpopulation of pygmy rabbits was geographically and genetically isolated in the Columbia Basin in central Washington State over 10,000 years ago. This population known as the Columbia Basin pygmy rabbit (CBPR) suffered a swift decline from 1995 to 2001 due to loss of their sagebrush habitat. Under emergency provisions, the CBPR was listed as endangered by the US Fish and Wildlife Service in November 2001.[1] Since that time, captive propagation attempts have been in progress at 3 facilities: Washington State University in Pullman, Washington; Oregon Zoo in Portland, Oregon; and Northwest Trek Wildlife Park in Eatonville, Washington.[2] These facilities recognized a high incidence of mycobacteriosis in captive CBPR, and in 2006 Harrenstien and collaborators performed a retrospective study in order to elucidate the clinical course of the disease, assess risk factors and to improve husbandry and medical management protocols.[3] This study confirmed disseminated mycobacteriosis due to *Mycobacterium avium* complex as

The author has nothing to disclose.
College of Veterinary Medicine, Western University of Health Sciences, 309 East Second Street, Pomona, CA 91766-1854, USA
E-mail address: dmcclure@westernu.edu

Vet Clin Exot Anim 15 (2012) 85–99
doi:10.1016/j.cvex.2011.11.002
1094-9194/12/$ – see front matter © 2012 Elsevier Inc. All rights reserved.

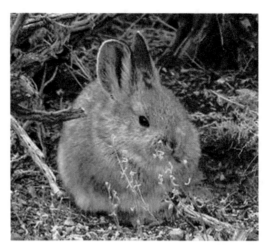

Fig. 1. The pygmy rabbit (*Brachylagus idahoensis*). (*From* Utah Conservation Data Center, Division of Wildlife Resources. Available at: http://dwrcdc.nr.utah.gov/rsgis2/Search/Display. asp?FlNm=bracidah.)

the most common cause of death in adult captive pygmy rabbits (29% of the captive adult population from June 2002 to September 2004; 37% of the captive adult from 2008 to 2011) regardless of origin.[2,3] Reports of mycobacteriosis in domestic rabbits (*Oryctolagus cuniculus*) are rare and have been associated with heavily contaminated *Mycobacterium bovis* or *M avium* subsp *paratuberculosis* cattle pasture.[4,5] It is believed that habitat fragmentation and geographic isolation led to inbreeding, which resulted in low genetic variation in the pygmy rabbit in the Columbia basin. This evolutionary bottleneck gave rise to the cell-mediated immunosuppression underlying the susceptibility of the CBPR to mycobacteriosis.

Healthy pygmy rabbits have been known to live longer than 4 years in captivity. The average onset of clinical signs later confirmed to be associated with mycobacteriosis

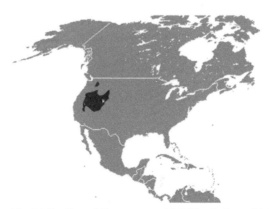

Fig. 2. The geographic distribution of the pygmy rabbit (*Brachylagus idahoensis*). (*Courtesy of* Chermundy and IUCN Red List of Threatened Species. *From:* http://commons.wikimedia. org/wiki/File:Pygmy_Rabbit_area.png.)

occurred at 28.5 months while the earliest onset was at 10.5 months of age. Mycobacteriosis occurred slightly more in females than in males. The clinical course is long and the clinical signs are nonspecific, including weight loss, lethargy, perineal soiling, and anorexia. An occasional presentation of lameness might be related to osteomyelitis. Clinical signs typical of mycobacteriosis in the pygmy rabbit and other mammalian species included pale mucous membranes due to anemia of chronic disease and dyspnea associated with granulomatous pneumonia. Lactation in non-pregnant rabbits (11% of cases) was a clinical finding unique to captive pygmy rabbits. Hematologic and biochemical findings were also nonspecific neutrophilia (most common finding), monocytosis, anemia, hypoalbuminemia, hyperglobulinemia, and/or hypercholesterolemia. Decreased albumin-globulin ratio was found in approximately 50% of serum biochemistry panels. Alkaline phosphatase elevation occurred in one animal with osteomyelitis.[2,3]

The antemortem diagnosis of respiratory mycobacteriosis can be made by the presence of abnormal respiratory sounds on thoracic auscultation, the presence of granulomas in lung or bone on a whole body radiograph. and reduced serum albumin-globulin ratio. Abdominal ultrasound was not useful to detect renal or hepatic granulomas. Presumptive confirmation includes acid-fast staining of cytologic preparations of aspirate or impression smears, culture, and serum/plasma antibody assays.[2,3] Mycobacterial cultures take weeks to complete and results may not be available until after death. Polymerase chain reaction (PCR) detection of *M avium* complex provides a much quicker diagnostic turnaround time.[2,6] Intradermal tuberculin testing has not been evaluated in pigmy rabbits.

Current captive population management includes routine postmortem collection of samples for histopathology and mycobacterial testing for any dead adult pygmy rabbit.[3] Histologic lesions include granulomatous inflammation, discrete granulomas, and necrotic foci. The Inflammatory response is predominantly macrophages with fewer neutrophils, lymphocytes, and plasma cells. Occasionally, inflammatory cells can be organized into discrete granulomas surrounding foci of caseous necrosis. Occasional Langhans-type multinucleate giant cells were present at the margin of necrotic tissue and inflammation in the granulomas.[3]

Due to the high incidence of mycobacteriosis in captive pygmy rabbit, therapeutic treatment should be initiated promptly as soon as a presumptive diagnosis has been made. A variety of treatment protocols have been attempted with limited success.[3] Current recommendations include empirical long-term treatment with a combination of azithromycin, rifabutin, and ethanbutol.[3]

Soil and water commonly contain *M avium* complex. As a burrowing species, the pygmy rabbit will routinely come in contact with this organism unless soil used in the enclosures is sterilized or eliminated. Other animal species should be excluded from pygmy rabbit housing as they could be potential sources of *M avium* complex.

Cell-mediated immunity was assessed using cytokine and lymphocyte stimulation assays.[3] The cytotoxic cellular response or the T helper 1 (Th1) response is necessary for an immune defense against mycobacteria. Pygmy rabbits produce lower concentrations of gamma-interferon, which would result in decreased macrophage activation and lower numbers of killer T cells. Pygmy rabbits also have elevated levels of T helper 2 (Th2) cytokines, which inhibit Th1 responses. These cytokine assay results suggest the pygmy rabbit Th1-Th2 response is unbalanced. The Th2 leads to disseminated mycobacteriosis, while the Th1 response is not present to protect against mycobacteria. There was a muted response to mitogen and major histocompatibility complex antigens in both the CBPR and Idaho pygmy rabbits. Intercrossing of CBPR with other nonendangered pygmy rabbit populations is being attempted to promote hybrid

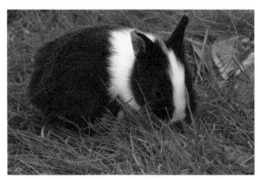

Fig. 3. A juvenile dwarf Netherland rabbit (*Oryctolagus cuniculus*). (*Courtesy of* color line. *From:* http://commons.wikimedia.org/wiki/File:Young_Netherland_Dwarf_rabbit.jpg.)

vigor. Thus far, the lymphocyte responses to antigens of intercrossed pygmy rabbits were similar to those of domestic rabbits, suggesting improvement in cell-mediated immunity and potential to lower incidence of disseminated mycobacteriosis in this species.[3]

There is one clinical case report of atypical mycobacterial infection confirmed in a juvenile dwarf rabbit (*Oryctolagus cuniculus*) (**Fig. 3**).[7] The patient presented with clinical signs of dyspnea and suspected ascites. The gross findings on necropsy included serosanguinous pleural effusion, whitish striated foci in the lungs, and multifocal scars in the cortex of the kidneys. Histopathology findings included severe granulomatous pneumonia with acid-fast bacteria; interstitial chronic lymphoplasma-cytic nephritis with interstitial fibrosis in the kidneys; and multifocal granulomatous and partly necrotizing encephalitis with microorganism suggestive of encephalitozoo-nosis.[7] *Mycobacterium genavense* was confirmed by PCR and 16S RNA gene sequencing. As the lungs were found to be the only affected organ, the authors suggested infection occurred through inhalation.

SPONTANEOUS MYCOBACTERIOSIS—RODENTS

There are few cases of spontaneous mycobacteriosis reported in pet rodents. In 1993, a colony of hairy-footed hamsters (*Phodopus sungorus*) (**Fig. 4**) was reported to have mycobacteriosis, which presented primarily with cutaneous lesions (ulcerative granulomatous dermatitis).[8] In 2007, disseminated mycobacteriosis was reported in a pet Korean squirrel (*Sciuris vulgaris coreae*) in Spain.[9] In 2009, a second case of mycobacteriosis in a pet squirrel was reported from the Iberian Peninsula. The second case involved a Richardson's ground squirrel (*Spermophilus richardsonii*) (**Fig. 5**) in Portugal.[10] Predominant findings in these squirrel cases included pulmonary lymph node, intestinal, and renal involvement confirmed on histopathology and acid-fast staining and positive PCR diagnostic tests. *M avium* subsp *avium* was identified in both squirrel cases. They presented similarly with less intestinal involvement in the Korean squirrel compared to the Richardson's ground squirrel. Ascites was described only in the Korean squirrel case. The source of infection was not identified for either case. The Richardson's ground squirrel was a male that was housed with 3 females for 3 months. The 3 exposed female squirrels remained negative for *Mycobacteria* by culture.

There are few cases of spontaneous mycobacteriosis reported in exotic rodents. Tuberculosis was reported in capybaras (*Hydrochoerus hydrochaeris*) (**Fig. 6**) in the Czech Republic, where *M bovis* was confirmed.[10] *Mycobacterium tuberculosis* was

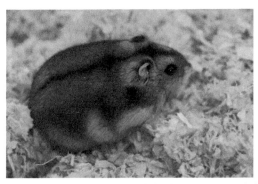

Fig. 4. The Djungarian or hairy-footed hamster (*Phodopus sungorus*). (*Courtesy of* Philipp Salzgeber, Wolfurt, Austria. *From:* http://commons.wikimedia.org/wiki/File:PhodopusSungorus_1.jpg.)

confirmed in an agouti from a Polish zoo.[11] At least 5 capybaras at the Basel Zoo in the period from 1956 to 1958 died due to tuberculosis caused by *M bovis*. These capybaras had been housed together with domestic ungulates.[12] A porcupine (specific species not stated) that had been transferred from Zurich to Basel Zoo in 1944 died 1 year later from tuberculosis.[12] From 1978 to 1982, a total of 16 common yellow-toothed cavies (*Galea musteloides*) died at Zurich zoos of pulmonary diseases. In some cases, acid-fast bacteria were identified, but bacterial identification was unsuccessful.[12]

Vole tuberculosis is the only spontaneous mycobacteriosis of clinical significance to rodents. Vole tuberculosis results in a chronic infection with severe pathology in its later stages. Vole tuberculosis affects the wild populations of field voles (*Microtus agrestis*) (**Fig. 7**), bank voles (*Clethrionomys glareolus*), wood mice (*Apodemus sylvaticus*), and shrews (*Sorex araneus*) in northern England, where it is an endemic disease.[13] The causative agent was first named *Mycobacterium tuberculosis* subsp

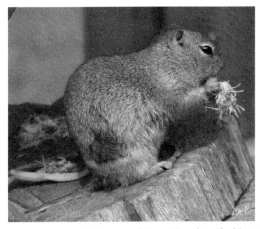

Fig. 5. Richardson's ground squirrel (*Spermophilus richardsonii*). (*Courtesy of* Dave Selby. *From:* http://commons.wikimedia.org/wiki/File:Richardson%27s_ground_squirrel.jpg.)

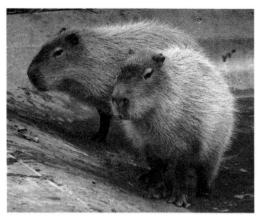

Fig. 6. Capybara (*Hydrochoerus hydrochaeris*). (*Courtesy of* Adrian Pingstone, Bristol, England. *From:* http://commons.wikimedia.org/wiki/File:Bristol.zoo.capybara.arp.jpg.)

muris and later *Mycobacterium microti*, which is a member of the *M. tuberculosis* complex.[14]

It was 60 years until this wild rodent disease became of interest once more when humans cases of *M microti* infection started to be reported in the late 1990s.[13,15] In the late 1990s, the Central Veterinary Laboratory compared the spoligotype patterns of *M tuberculosis* complex strains in its database with an international database at the National Institute of Public Health and the Environment in the Netherlands. The patterns of 11 *M tuberculosis* complex isolates were identical of highly similar to the spoligotypes of *M microti* isolates. One of these isolates was from a human.[16] The identification of *M microti* infections had been hampered by the very slow growth of the organism in vitro. It takes 4 weeks to growth *M bovis*, but *M microti* takes 8 weeks. Comparing additional *M tuberculosis* complex databases revealed additional human *M microti* infections involving both immunocompetent and immunocompromised humans.[16] Three spoligotypes of *M microti* have been identified: vole, llama, and Dassie rock hyrax types.[13] The vole and llama types have been found in the Netherlands, Belgium, the United Kingdom, and France.[13] The Dassie rock hyrax type

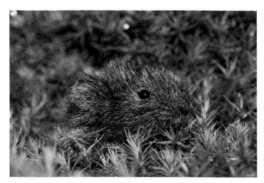

Fig. 7. The field vole (*Microtus agrestis*). (*Courtesy of* Fer Boei, Kaapse Bossen, Utrecht, Netherlands. *From:* http://commons.wikimedia.org/wiki/File:Aardmuis.jpg.)

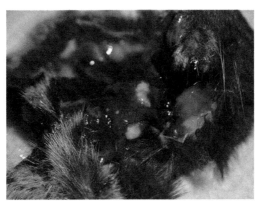

Fig. 8. Internal pathologic tuberculosis lesions of voles includes multiple cream-colored caseous abscesses under the skin and in the abdomen. (*Courtesy of* Malcolm Bennett, BVSc, PhD, MRCVS, FRCPath, FHEA, Liverpool, UK.)

was isolated in South African Dassie rock hyrax after being imported to the Perth Zoo and a Canadian zoo.[17–19] Zoonotic infection with *M microti* has been recorded in immunosuppressed and immunocompetent humans.[15,16,20,21]

Although the optimal diagnosis would be detection of *M microti* in urine or feces, researchers failed to find the organism when using spoligotyping in voles with clinical signs of disease.[13] Prevalence determination based on postmortem identification of internal pathologic tuberculosis lesions was 21% compared to a prevalence of 7% when based on external clinical signs alone.[13,22] Internal lesions described as obvious lymphadenitis, multiple tuberculous lesions (cream-colored caseous abscesses) under the skin and in the abdomen (**Fig. 8**) and pulmonary granulomas (**Fig. 9**).

More recently, researchers studied several populations in the Kielder Forest, UK, in order to understand the effect of vole tuberculosis on the field vole (*Microtus agrestis*).[23] The prevalence of the disease ranged from 0% to 50% depending on the

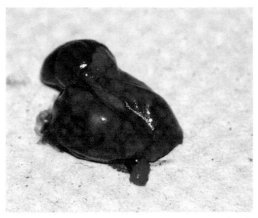

Fig. 9. Lung with multiple pulmonary tubercular lesions in a vole. (*Courtesy of* Malcolm Bennett, BVSc, PhD, MRCVS, FRCPath, FHEA, Liverpool, UK.)

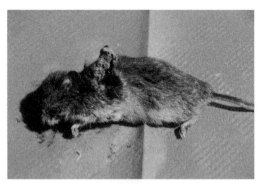

Fig. 10. Carcass of a vole with external skin lesion typical of vole tuberculosis. (*Courtesy of* Malcolm Bennett, BVSc, PhD, MRCVS, FRCPath, FHEA, Liverpool, UK.)

site study: 5.2% of animals had observable lesions, while 10.78% were found to be positive for *M microti* organisms. The disease prevalence varied with the age of the animals. The disease prevalence (13.15%) was also higher in the springtime. The seasonality is likely related to the increased numbers of older voles that were present in the population in the springtime. The advanced stages of the disease were more prevalent in older animals and were external lesions were seen only on animals greater than 17 g. The appearance of cutaneous lesions was correlated with advanced disease (**Fig. 10**). Body condition score diminished after lesions were observed, which suggests an acute phase of infection during advanced stages of the disease. The predicted survival following the appearance of a cutaneous lesion was not significantly different from that of uninfected individuals.[23]

The Institute of Zoology of the Cuban Academy of Science described 2 types of mycobacteriosis (*M tuberculosis* and *M avium-intracellulare* complex) in 2 specimens of Cuban tree rat or Hutia (*Capromys pilorides*) (**Fig. 11**).[24]

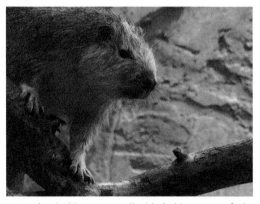

Fig. 11. Cuban tree rat or hutia (*Capromys pilorides*). (*Courtesy of* Alena Houšková, Děčín, Czech Republic. *From:* http://commons.wikimedia.org/wiki/File:Hutia-konga_Capromys_pilorides_ZOO_D%C4%9B%C4%8D%C3%ADn.jpg.)

INDUCED MYCOBACTERIOSIS—RABBITS AND RODENTS

Although rabbits and rodents are not susceptible to mycobacteriosis, they have played an important role as animal models to study the pathogenesis of tuberculosis and other mycobacteriosis and for development of diagnostics tests, vaccines, and other therapeutic treatments used to battle mycobacterial disease.[25–33] The guinea pig, rabbit, and nonhuman primate develop cavitary pulmonary disease similar to humans.[30,31] The key feature is development of necrotic central lesions. These are associated with alterations in physiologic functions such as the development of hypoxia.[34] The rabbit will also develop extrapulmonary dissemination of *M bovis* and not *M tuberculosis*.[25] While the rabbit has been a leading model of mycobacterial pathogenesis, the guinea pig has been the gold standard for the development of vaccines.[29] Disease severity in the guinea pig is a useful virulence measure. From the Wistar rat to the Beige/Scid (immunodeficient) mouse, rats and mice have been valuable models in a variety of contexts. They have been particular useful revealing the details of the immune response to mycobacteria and the role of the routes of infection and parsing out antibiotic treatment protocols.[30,33]

RABBITS AND RODENTS AS WILDLIFE RESERVOIRS FOR *MYCOBACTERIUM*

North America, Europe, and New Zealand are at the risk for tuberculosis and tuberculosis is a potential reemerging disease at the wildlife–domestic animal interface.[35–38] *M bovis* is a concern for agricultural livestock species. Increasing anthropogenic factors such as translocation of wildlife, supplemental feeding of wildlife by the public, and altered wildlife population densities are increasing the risk for zoonosis and returning infection to domestic livestock populations. A variety of wild mammalian species have been targeted as having a role in tuberculosis epidemiology. The epidemiology at *M bovis* involving wild mammals and domestic lifestock has been outlined in the following systems:

- In Australia—the feral pig (*Sus scrofa*); the feral Asian water buffalo (*Bubalus bubalis*)[36,37]
- In Michigan—the white tailed deer (*Odocoileus virginianus*)[36,37]
- In New Zealand—the brushtail opossum (*Trichosurus vulpecula*); the ferret (*Mustela furo*)[36,37]
- In the United Kingdom—the European badger (*Meles meles*)[36,37,39,40]
- In Canada—the wood bison (*Bison bison antabascae*) in/around Wood Buffalo National Park; the wapiti (*Cervus elaphus manitobensis*) in/around the Riding Mountain National Park.[41,42]

The potential of rabbits and rodents as a reservoir for *Mycobacterium* spp has not been fully explored. There is a lack of surveillance data and it is not possible to rule out deep population of mammals in their role in the epidemiology of tuberculosis. *M bovis* and *M avium* complex has been isolated from rodent species. Wells and Oxen first reported *Mycobacterium* spp in rodents in 1937.[43] They reported a prevalence of *Mycobacterium microti* between 9% and 31% in rodents. In 1946, mycobacteria were isolated from the lung, spleen, liver, kidney, and lymph nodes in 1.6% of tuberculosis lesions of 8 of 500 shrews caught in Great Britain.[44] Additional details regarding *M microti* were discussed earlier in this article.

More recently, some wild rodent populations have been evaluated for *M bovis*. Considering the widespread cattle and badger tuberculosis infection known in south Dorset, England, wild rats (*Rattus norvegicus*) were investigated as a possible wild rodent reservoir of *M bovis*. *M bovis* was not found in the rat and this led to the

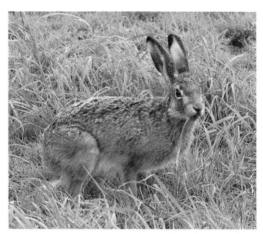

Fig. 12. European brown hare (*Lepus europaeus*). (*Courtesy of* MOdmate, Schiermonnikoog, Netherlands. *From:* http://en.wikipedia.org/wiki/File:Feldhase_Schiermonnikoog.JPG.)

conclusion that the badger was the only wild mammal reservoir.[45] *M bovis* was found in 5% of hedgehogs and 0.6% to 2.8% of rodents in the southwest region of England. One study in a German wild animal park monitored several sentinel species during an ongoing tuberculosis (*M bovis)* outbreak in cattle.[42] Human caretakers, silver fox (*Vulpes vulpes*), European badger (*Meles meles*), ferret (*Mustela furo*), and rodents (specific rodent species were not identified) were monitored for *M bovis* from 2000 to 2006. All monitored sentinel species remained negative for *M bovis*.[42]

The first suspected case of *M avium* subsp *paratuberculosis* in a European brown hare (*Lepus europaeus*) (**Fig. 12**) was reported in England in 1977.[46] In 1990, lesions attributed to paratuberculosis were described in a wild rabbit (**Fig. 13**) in Scotland.[47] As paratuberculosis or Johne's disease results in fatal enteritis in all ruminants, it is associated with economic losses in domestic livestock. Investigations of paratuberculosis in Scotland have extended into surveillance of nonruminant wild populations.

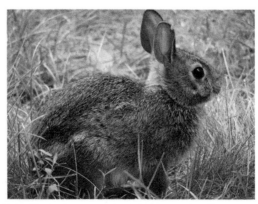

Fig. 13. A wild rabbit (*Oryctolagus cuniculus*). (*Courtesy of* EIC. *From:* http://commons.wikimedia.org/wiki/File:Rabbit-closeup-profile.jpg.)

Three surveys of rabbits from farms in eastern Scotland confirmed paratuberculosis by postmortem signs of thicken bowels and lymphadenopathy and then by histopathology and positive cultures.[48–50] A wild rabbit isolate was able to infect calves experimentally.[51] As paratuberculosis is notoriously difficult to control, it was suggested that nonruminant wildlife reservoirs of paratuberculosis might be to blame. A statistically significant relationship between rabbit paratuberculosis and farms with previous or current paratuberculosis has been found.[49] The potential risk from wildlife has been reviewed.[4] Species other than rabbits were included in the review. This investigation concluded that granivorous or omnivorous rodents are likely to be infected from contaminated livestock feces. Rodents trapped in livestock housing had a higher prevalence of *M avium* subsp *paratuberculosis* than rodents captured in field margins or woodlands. The overall prevalence (62%) was greater for predators (foxes, stoats, and weasels) than that (10%) for prey species (rabbits, rats, and wood mice). Corvids play a double role as they can be infected by eating infected carrion and are a source of infection for predators.[52]

The rabbit is thought to pose the greatest risk to cattle due to the high concentration of mycobacterium in rabbit fecal pellets (10^6 CFU/g feces) and because cattle do not avoid eating rabbit fecal material while grazing.[53] A field study aimed to determine the modes of transmission of *M avium* subsp *paratuberculosis* within wild rabbit populations in Scotland and whether the infection could be maintained suggested that *M avium* subsp *paratuberculosis* could be transmitted vertically (transplacental), pseudo-vertically (from contaminated milk/or feces), and horizontally.[54] Of offspring entering the population of rabbits at 1 month of age, 14% were positive. As the organism is very slow growing, the prevalence at 1 month underestimates the true prevalence. The actual prevalence of the infection may be as high as 46%. The data suggest horizontal transmission is probable over the 18-month life span of the wild rabbit. The probability of these 3 modes of transmission indicates that *M avium* subsp. *paratuberculosis* could be maintained in the wild rabbit population.[54]

In North America, the potential role has been evaluated of wild rabbits and deer as sources of *M avium* subsp *paratuberculosis* for Minnesota Dairy herds.[55] In this study, the prevalence of *M avium* subsp *paratuberculosis* in rabbit or deer feces was low (2% and 4%, respectively). The primary risk was for the rabbits and deer from cattle and not for cattle from rabbits or deer. In fact, farms practices, such as using a common calving pen or by using pooled colostrums, were more significant in the transmission of infection. Other farm practices such as manure spreading on crop fields or pasture increase the spread of infection to deer and rabbits.

Developing countries have growing numbers of immunocompromised human populations, one cause being the spread of HIV/AIDS.[38] This fact is making detection and surveillance of mycobacteria in rodents and insectivores increasing concerns. In 2008, Durnez and collaborators were the first to report findings of mycobacteria in African rodents and insectivores[38]; 2.65% of the trapped animals were carriers of mycobacteria (including *M avium* complex). There was a higher prevalence of mycobacteria in urban areas than in the field environment. Nontuberculous mycobacteria (*M chimaera*, *M intracellulare*, *M arupanse*, *M parascrofulaceum*, and *Mycobacterium* spp) were isolated from the Gambian pouched rat (*Cricetomys gambianus*) (**Fig. 14**), Multimammate rat or the African soft-furred rat (*Mastomus natalensis*), and the insectivorous lesser red musk shrew (*Crocidura hirta*). This was the first study to use stratified pool screening and mycobacterial ecology to estimate prevalence, thus demonstrating that detection of *Mycobacterium* spp in these animals is more effective than environmental surveillance. The report did not present evidence that rodents are serving as reservoirs for mycobacteria, and further studies

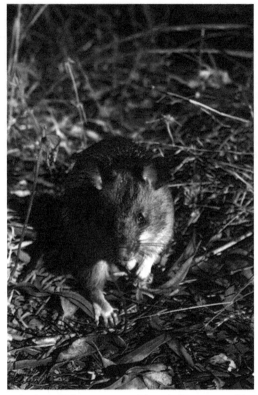

Fig. 14. Gambian pouched rat (*Cricetomys gambianus*). (*Courtesy of* Derek Keats, Johannesburg, South Africa. *From:* http://commons.wikimedia.org/wiki/File:Afr-giant-rat.jpg.)

on the presence of mycobacteria in rodent feces are under way. Several ways of transmission of mycobacteria are possible: through direct contact with rodent feces, ingestion of food or water contaminated with rodent excreta, ingestion of the animal itself, and through inhaling aerosolized fecal material. Potentially pathogenic mycobacteria are found in rodents and they could impact the health of other animals or immunocompromised humans.

SUMMARY

Spontaneous mycobacteriosis is rare in rabbits and rodents with the exception of the pygmy rabbit; there are only a handful of reported cases involving hairy-footed hamsters, a pet Korean squirrel, and a Richardson's ground squirrel. The susceptibility of the pygmy rabbit to lethal disseminating mycobacteriosis is a result of underlying cell-mediated immune function deficiency. In all reports of spontaneous mycobacteriosis involving rabbits and rodents, *M avium* complex was identified. The resistance of rabbits and rodents to mycobacterial disease has been useful in understanding the disease in humans and animals. The measures taken to defeat the rabbit or rodent immune system to induce mycobacteriosis have provided useful insight to a complex pathophysiology and ecology. While rabbits and rodents are resistant to disease, they do have the potential to carry or transmit mycobacteria within the environment and to people and animals. Preventing or controlling *Mycobacterium* sp transmission wildlife to domestic animals will require collaboration between agriculture, wildlife, environmental, and political entities. Understanding the ecology and epidemiology of mycobacteria is needed for better worldwide management of tuberculosis.

REFERENCES

1. Hays DW. Washington pygmy rabbit emergency action plan for species survival: addendum to Washington State Recovery Plan for the Pygmy Rabbit (1995). Available at: http://wdfw.wa.gov/publications/pub.php?id=00277. Accessed August 2001.
2. Harrenstien LA, Finnegan M, Case A, et al. Disease issues affecting species recovery of the Columbia Basin pygmy rabbit (*Brachylagus idahoensis*). Presented at the Association of Avian Veterinarians 32nd Annual Conference and Expo with the Association of Exotic Mammal Veterinarians. Seattle, August 6-12, 2011. p. 433–8.
3. Harrenstien LA, Finnegan MV, Woodford NL, et al. *Mycobacterium avium* in pygmy rabbits (*Brachylagus idahoensis*): 28 cases. J Zoo Wildl Med 2006;37:498–512.
4. Daniels MJ, Hutchings MR, Beard MP, et al. Do non-ruminant wildlife pose a risk of paratuberculosis to domestic livestock and vice versa in Scotland? J Wildl Dis 2003;39:10–5.
5. Hines ME 2nd, Kreeger KJ, Herron AJ, et al. Mycobacterial infections of animals: pathology and pathogenesis. Lab Anim Sci 1995;45:334–51.
6. Iralu JV, Sritharan VK, Vieciak PS, et al. Diagnosis of *Mycobacterium avium* bacteremia by polymerase chain reaction. J Clin Microbiol 1993;31:1811–4.
7. Ludwig E, Reischl U, Janik D, et al: Granulomatous Pneumonia Caused by *Mycobacterium genavense* in a Dwarf rabbit (*Oryctolagus cuniculus*). Vet Pathol 2009;46: 1000–2.
8. Martinez MJ, Nichols DK, et al. Mycobacteriosis in hairy-footed hamsters (*Phodopus sungorus*). In: Proceedings of the American Association of Zoo Veterinarians Annual Conference. St. Louis (MO), October 9-14, 1993. p. 346.
9. Moreno B, Aduriz G, Garrido JM, et al. Disseminated *Mycobacterium avium* subsp. *avium* infection in a pet Korean squirrel (*Sciurus vulgaris coreae*). Vet Pathol 2007;44: 123–5.
10. Juan-Sallés C, Patricio R, Garrido J, et al. Disseminated *Mycobacterium avium* subsp. *avium* infection in a captive Richardson's ground squirrel (*Spermophilus richardsonii*). J Exot Pet Med 2009;18:306–10.
11. Pavlik I, Yayo AW, Parmova I, et al. *Mycobacterium tuberculosis* in animal and human populations in six Central European countries during 1990-1999. Vet Med 2003;48: 83–9.
12. Dollinger P, Baumgartner R, Isenbügel E, et al. Husbandry and pathology of rodent and logon works in Swiss zoos. Verh Ber Erkg Zoot 1999:39.
13. Cavanagh R, Begon M, Bennett M, et al. *Mycobacterium microti* infection (vole tuberculosis) in wild rodent populations. J Clin Microbiol 2002;40:3281–5.
14. Brooke WS. The vole acid-fast bacillus. Am Rev Tuberc 1941;43:806–16.
15. Kremer K, van Soolingen D, van Embden J, et al. *Mycobacterium microti*: more widespread than previously thought. J Clin Microbiol 1998;36:2793–4.
16. van Soolingen D, van der Zanden AGM, de Haas PEW, et al. Diagnosis of *Mycobacterium microti* infections among humans by using novel genetic markers. J Clin Microbiol 1998;36:1840–5.
17. Cousins DV, Gaynor PR, Williams SN, et al. Tuberculosis in imported hyrax (*Procavia capensis*) caused by an unusual variant belonging to the *Mycobacterium tuberculosis* complex. Vet Microbiol 1994;42:135–45.

18. Lutze-Wallace C, Turcotte C, Glover D, et al.: Isolation of *Mycobacterium microti*-like organism from a rock hyrax (*Procavia capensis*) in a Canadian zoo. Can Vet J 2006;47:1011–3.
19. Smith N. The dassie' bacillus. Tubercle 1990;41:203–12.
20. Niemann S, Richter E, Dalugge-Tamm H, et al. Two cases of *Mycobacterium microti*-derived tuberculosis in HIV-negative immunocompetent patients. Emerg Infect Dis 2000;6:539–42.
21. Horstkotte MA, Sobottka I, Schewe CK, et al. *Mycobacterium microti* llama-type infection presenting as pulmonary tuberculosis in a human immunodeficiency virus-positive patient. J Clin Microbiol 2001;39:406–7.
22. Cavanagh R, Lambin X, Ergon T, et al. Disease dynamics in cyclic populations of field voles (*Microtus agrestis*): cowpox virus and vole tuberculosis (*Mycobacterium microti*). Proceedings of the Royal Society of London, B 2004;271:859–67.
23. Burthe S, Kipar Bm, Lambin A. Tuberculosis (*Mycobacterium microti*) in wild field vole populations. Parasitology 2008;135:309–17.
24. Cornide R, Ferra C, Jimenez C, et al. Hallazgo de *Mycobacterium* (*M tuberculosis* and *avium-intracellulare* complex) in *Capromys pilorides*. Rev Cub Cienc Vet 1989;20: 199–202.
25. Flynn JL, Cooper A, Bishai WR. Animal models of tuberculosis. In: Cole ST, Eisenach KD, McMurray DN, Jacobs WR, editors. Tuberculosis and the tubercle bacillus. Washington, DC: ASM Press; 2005. p. 547–60.
26. Dharmadhikari AS, Nardell EA: What animal models teach humans about tuberculosis. Am J Respir Cell Mol Biol 2008;39:503–8.
27. Bishai WR. Extrapulmonary dissemination of *Mycobacterium bovis* but not *Mycobacterium tuberculosis* in a bronchoscopic rabbit model of cavitary tuberculosis. Infect Immun 2009;77:598–603.
28. North RJ. *Mycobacterium tuberculosis* is strikingly more virulent for mice when given via the respiratory than via the intravenous route. J Infect Dis 1995;172:1550–3.
29. Orme IM. Preclinical testing of new vaccines for tuberculosis: a comprehensive review. Vaccine 2006;24:2–19.
30. Orme IM, McMurray DN. The immune response to tuberculosis in animal models. In: Rom WN, Garay S, editors. Tuberculosis. Boston (MA): Little, Brown; 1996.
31. Palanisamy GS, Smith EE, Shanley CA, et al. Disseminated disease severity as a measure of virulence of Mycobacterium tuberculosis in the guinea pig model. Tuberculosis 2008;88:295–306.
32. Seiler P, Aichele P, Bandermann S, et al: Early granuloma formation after aerosol *Mycobacterium tuberculosis* infection is regulated by neutrophils via CXCR3-signaling chemokines. Eur J Immunol 2003;33:2676–86.
33. Young D. Animal models of tuberculosis Eur J Immunol 2009;39:2011–4.
34. Via LE, Lin PL, Ray SM, et al: Tuberculous granulomas are hypoxic in guinea pigs, rabbits, and nonhuman primates. Infect Immun 2008;76:2333–40.
35. Biet F, Boschiroli ML, Thorel MFo, et al. Zoonotic aspects of *Mycobacterium bovis* and *Mycobacterium avium-intracellulare* complex (MAC). Vet Res 2005;36:411–36.
36. Corner L. The role of wild animal populations in the epidemiology of tuberculosis in domestic animals: how to assess the risk. Vet Microbiol 2006;112:303–12.
37. Palmer MV. Tuberculosis: a reemerging disease at the interface of domestic animals and wildlife. Curr Top Microbiol Immunol 2007;315:195–215.
38. Lies-Durnez ME, Mgode GF, Katakweba A, et al. First detection of Mycobacteria in African Rodents and insectivores using stratified pool screening. App Env Microbiol 2008;74:768–73.

39. Smith GC. Models of *Mycobacterium bovis* in wildlife and cattle. Tuberculosis 2001; 81:51–64.
40. Delahay RJ, Barlow AM, Walker N, et al. Bovine tuberculosis infection in wild mammals in the South-West region of England: a survey of prevalence and a semi-quantitative assessment of the relative risks to cattle. Vet J 2007;173:287–301.
41. Nishi JS, Shury T, Elkin BT. Wildlife reservoirs for bovine tuberculosis (*Mycobacterium bovis*) in Canada: strategies for management and research. Vet Microbiol 2006;112: 325–38.
42. Schmidbauer SM, Wohlsein P, Kirpal G, et al. Outbreak of *Mycobacterium bovis* infection in a wild animal park. Vet Rec 2007;161:304–7.
43. Wells AQ, Oxon DM. Tuberculosis in wild voles. Lancet 1937;1:1221.
44. Lapage G. Tuberculosis of voles and shrews. Nature 1947;160:168.
45. Little T, C Swan, HV Thompson, et al. Bovine tuberculosis in domestic and wild mammals in an area of Dorset. III. The prevalence of tuberculosis in mammals other than badgers and cattle. J Hygiene 1982;89:225–34.
46. Mathews PR, Sargent A. The isolation of mycobacteria from the brown Hare (*Lepus europaeus*). Brit Vet J 1977;133:399–404.
47. Angus K. Intestinal lesions resembling paratuberculosis in a wild rabbit (*Oryctolagus cuniculus*). J Comp Pathol 1990;103:22–3.
48. Greig A, Stevenson K, Perez V, et al. Paratuberculosis in wild rabbits (*Oryctolagus cuniculus*). Vet Rec 1997;140:141–3.
49. Greig A, Stevenson K, Henderson D, et al. Epidemiological study of paratuberculosis in wild rabbits in Scotland. J Clin Microbiol 1999;37:1746–51.
50. Beard, PM, Rhind SM, Buxton D, et al. Natural paratuberculosis infection in rabbits in Scotland. J Comp Pathol 2001;124:290–9.
51. Beard PM, Stevenson K, Pirie A, et al. Experimental paratuberculosis in calves following inoculation with a rabbit isolate of Mycobacterium avium subsp. paratuberculosis. J Clin Microbiol 2001;39:3080–4.
52. Beard PM,Daniels MJ, Henderson D. Paratuberculosis infection of nonruminant wildlife in Scotland. Clin Microbiol 2001;39:1517–21.
53. Judge J, Greig A, Kyriazakis I, et al. Ingestion of faeces by grazing herbivores-risk of inter-species disease transmission. Agric Ecosyst Environ 2005;107:267–74.
54. Judge J, Kyriazakis I, Greig A, et al: Routes of intraspecies transmission of *Mycobacterium avium* subsp. *paratuberculosis* in rabbits (*Oryctolagus cuniculus*): a field study. Appl Envir Microbiol 2006;72:398–403.
55. Raizman, EA. *Mycobacterium avium* supsp. *paratuberculosis* from free-ranging deer and rabbits surrounding Minnesota dairy herds. Michigan Bovine Tuberculosis Bibliography and Database. Fort Collins (CO): National Wildlife Research Center, USDA/APHIS/Wildlife Services; 2005. Available at: http://digitalcommons.unl.edu/michbo vinetb. Accessed November 17, 2011.

Mycobacterial Infections in Reptiles

Mark A. Mitchell, DVM, MS, PhD, DECZM (Herpetology)

KEYWORDS

- Granulomatous • *Mycobacteria* • Mycobacteriosis
- Reptiles • Zoonoses

Mycobacteria represent an interesting group of bacteria. These slow-growing, slender, aerobic, acid-fast, Gram-positive rods have a long history in human medicine. Known to cause the devastating diseases associated with tuberculosis and leprosy, affected individuals were once separated from society because of the concerns associated with contagion. Although there has been a great deal of study associated with these pathogens in humans, there has been much less in animals, especially reptiles.

Current thought suggests that veterinarians working with exotic animals are much more likely to encounter cases of mycobacteriosis in birds and fish than in reptiles. The differences noted between groups may be attributed to the fact that some of these organisms are better suited to survive in endotherms (eg, humans, birds); however, there are certainly a number of mycobacteria that thrive better in cooler temperatures (*Mycobacterium marinum* in fish). Because reptiles are ectotherms, but have the potential to achieve body temperatures on par or higher than endotherms through basking, it is possible that their role in the epidemiology of *Mycobacterium* spp infections may be greater than currently represented. A major shortcoming of measuring the prevalence of mycobacteria in reptiles can be associated with a lack of follow through with postmortem diagnosis and diagnostic testing. Although the author has seen a number of reptile cases over the years presented for diseases of a chronic nature, follow through on these cases with complete antemortem or postmortem examinations has been limited by financial constraints of the client. Is it possible that some of these cases would be confirmed as mycobacteriosis? It may be true; however, this question can be answered only if veterinary clinicians can fully pursue these types of cases with the appropriate diagnostic tests and postmortem evaluations. Ultimately, whether these cases are associated with mycobacteriosis or not, follow through with cases will help to better refine the evidence-based literature on which we depend.

The purpose of this article is to review the literature as it relates to mycobacteriosis in reptiles. Knowledge of the epidemiology of this disease can be useful to

The author has nothing to disclose.
Department of Veterinary Clinical Medicine, College of Veterinary Medicine, University of Illinois, 1008 West Hazelwood Drive, Urbana, IL 61802, USA
E-mail address: mmitch@illinois.edu

veterinarians working with these animals, especially when working on a diagnosis and making recommendations to clients.

MYCOBACTERIAL INFECTIONS IN CROCODILIANS

There are 23 different species of crocodilians, and *Mycobacterium* spp, or *Mycobacterium*-like lesions, have been described in at least 26% (6/23) of these animals.[1–5] This should not, however, be surprising because these animals live in an aquatic medium that is quite capable of harboring *Mycobacterium* spp. It is likely that other species of crocodilians have likewise been exposed but not reported.[2] Crocodilians that do develop mycobacteriosis tend to develop lesions in the respiratory, integumentary, and gastrointestinal systems.[2–5]

Mycobacterium or *Mycobacterium*-like organisms are most often found in farm-raised crocodilians.[1,3,6] Again, this too should not be surprising because these facilities tend to have higher than normal stocking densities, organic enriched water, and the crocodilians are under some degree of stress because of these conditions. Nevarez reported seeing acid-fast organisms consistent with *Mycobacterium* sp in captive American alligators (*Alligator mississipiensis*) (**Table 1**).[3] The animals originally presented for pneumonia and had 1–4 mm focal white lesions in the lungs. Granulomatous pneumonia has also been reported in farm-raised *Crocodylus johnstoni, C niloticus,* and *C porosus* in Africa, Australia, and Asia. It is unknown if age has a protective role against infection, as both young *C johnstoni* and at least one older animal (25 years old) have been found to develop clinical disease (see **Table 1**).[5,7] A review of the literature might suggest that younger animals are more susceptible, but it is important to recognize that there is an age bias in animals held in captivity for production of leather and meat, with young animals being the primary cohort. Although most frequently reported in captive animals raised in production facilities, there are also cases of pet animals developing the disease.[2]

In many parts of the world crocodilians serve as an important production species because of the value of their leather (Africa, Asia, Australia, and the United States). In some places, these animals may also serve as an important protein source or a novelty food.[8] Because these animals are handled or consumed, and they have been found to harbor *Mycobacterium* sp or *Mycobacterium*-like species, it is important to consider the potential role they may play in disseminating zoonotic pathogens to their caretakers. Exposure via consumptions should be minimal, as overall prevalence would be expected to be low.[8] Exposure via direct contact may be more likely depending on the types of practices/exposures an individual has with the aquatic environment and the crocodilians. Caretakers' health status may also influence their risk. There are certainly species of *Mycobacterium* that have been isolated from both crocodiles and humans, and thus there is the potential that the organisms can grow in both species. For example, *M szulgai* has been reported in at least 24 human cases.[9] This organism is typically found in pulmonary lesions in humans, but has also been found in joint lesions. This organism was also recently reported in a *C johnstoni* with granulomatous pneumonia (see **Table 1**).[5] *M marinum* is another common aquatic form of mycobacteria that is commonly thought to be a pathogen of poikilotherms, such as fish and reptiles (including crocodilians), but has also been reported in humans (eg, fisherman's finger, swimming pool granuloma).[1]

It is likely that direct contact with contaminated water or crocodilian skin would be the greatest source of exposure to humans. One study reported that the prevalence of *Mycobacterium*-like organisms in the skin of saltwater crocodiles (*C porosus*) was low (2.5%).[6] Fortunately, the reports associated with mycobacteriosis in crocodilians are rare; however, when individuals are working with these animals they may be

Table 1

Mycobacterium spp isolated from reptiles under natural or experimental conditions

Group	Reptile sp	Mycobacterium sp	Site of Infection	Exp/Nat Infection
Crocodilians	*Alligator mississipiensis*	*Mycobacterium* sp	Respiratory	Natural
	Caiman crocodilus fuscus	*M chelonae*	Respiratory	Natural
		M szulgai	Hepatic	
	Caiman crocodiles	*M marinum*		Natural
		M fortuitum		
	Crocodylus johnstoni	*M szulgai*	Respiratory	Natural
	Crocodylus niloticus	*Mycobacterium* sp	Respiratory	Natural
			Integument	
	Crocodylus porosus	*Mycobacterium* sp	Integument	Natural
Lizard	*Anolis carolinensis*	*M ulcerans*	Subcutaneous, gastrointestinal, hepatic	Experimental
	Chlamydosaurus kingi		Myocarditis, systemic	Natural
	Pogona vitticeps	*M marinum*	Pulmonary, joints	Natural
	Uromastyx aegypticus	*M marinum*	Joints	Natural
Snakes	*Boa constrictor*		Systemic	Natural (Kiel)
	Boa constrictor		Stomatitis	Natural
	Elaphe quadrivitta	*M leprae*	Systemic	Experimental
	Python regius	*M haemophilum*	Pulmonary	Natural (Div.)
		M marinum		
Turtles	*Apalone spinifera spinifera*	*M chelonae*	Intravascular	Natural
	Chelonia mydas	*M avium*	Pulmonary	Natural
	Chelodina Longicollis	*M marinum*	Systemic	Natural
	Lepidochelys kempii	*M chelonae*	Bone, joint, liver, kidney, lung, spleen, pericardium	Natural
	Kinosternon leukostonum	*M lepraemurium*	Liver	Experimental
	Pelodiscus sinensis	*M kansasii*		Natural
	Phrynops hilari	*Mycobacterium* sp	Cutaneous, liver, spleen,	Natural
	Terrapene carolina carolina	*M terrae*	Cutaneous, systemic	Natural

performing activities that increase their risk for exposure. For example, individuals responsible for removing the leather from these animals after euthanasia may be more likely to injure themselves when working with a sharp knife or have previous unhealed cuts that could serve as a source for exposure to *Mycobacterium* spp in the water or on the animal. Individuals charged with these higher risk activities should wear gloves and protect any small lacerations or abrasions on their hands with appropriate bandage material to minimize their exposure. Also, individuals working in aquatic systems with captive crocodilians should routinely wash their hands to minimize their exposure to these ubiquitous organisms.

Crocodilians are most likely exposed to *Mycobacterium* spp. via horizontal routes: contaminated water and food. The species isolated from crocodilians, including *M fortuitum*, *M marinum*, *M fuscus*, and *M szulgai*, are all common aquatic inhabitants and are also found in fish and other species of vertebrates commonly eaten by crocodilians.[1,2] The recent reports of *M. szulgai* in a freshwater crocodile (*C johnstoni*) and a brown caiman (*Caiman crocodilus fuscus*) from Korea and the Czech Republic, respectively, should reinforce the ubiquitous nature of these organisms (see **Table 1**).[2,5]

MYCOBACTERIAL INFECTIONS IN LIZARDS

There have been at least five reports of naturally occurring mycobacteriosis cases in lizards: a water monitor (*Varanus semirenex*), Egyptian spiny tailed lizards (*Uromastyx aegypticus*), a frilled lizard (*Chlamydosaurus kingi*), and two bearded dragons (*Pogona vitticeps*) (see **Table 1**).[10–14]

The case of mycobacteriosis in a (presumed) wild caught water monitor was described in Australia.[10] The animal did not adapt to captivity and was euthanized because of its poor condition. On postmortem examination the animal was emaciated and had 2- to 10-mm nodules throughout the viscera. Histopathologic examination of the lesions noted an inflammatory response; the tissues were acid fast negative by the Ziehl-Neelsen method but positive by the auramine fluorescent method. Eventually, *M intracellulare* was isolated from culture and inoculation into a live chicken. This pathogen is of interest because it is associated with human disease. Although it is certainly found in the soil and aquatic environments, its ability to grow in an ectotherm, such as the monitor lizard, while infecting humans, suggests that infected reptiles could serve as a reservoir or source of exposure for humans working with them. Special care should be taken when working with reptiles presenting with signs consistent with mycobacteriosis to minimize potential human exposure.

A case of mycobacteriosis associated with *M marinum*, a common fish pathogen, was described in a group of *Uromastyx* spp.[14] The animals were confiscated and designated to a zoological institution. The animals did poorly during the time they were in captivity. Lesions noted on the animals were associated primarily with the skin and toes. Because this pathogen is common in aquatic environments and grows best at cooler temperatures, it was suspected that the distribution of lesions was attributed to the cooler temperatures of the extremities. Similar descriptions can be found in humans.

The case of the mycobacteriosis in the frilled lizard (*Chlamydosaurus kingi*) was associated with a systemic illness.[12] This case should demonstrate that reptiles may present for clinical disease associated with organ dysfunction, not necessarily considered to be infections (eg, cardiac disease), and that a complete workup is required to confirm the cause of disease. In this particular animal, managing cardiac failure alone would have eventually had poor results.

The recent case reports of mycobacteriosis in bearded dragons are important, as these animals are extremely popular pets in the United States and Europe. Many of these animals are kept in households with children, and thus the zoonotic concern becomes more important because this population is less likely to appreciate the importance of practicing good hygiene and disinfection after handling their pet reptiles. This was well documented during the 1970s in the United States with the reports of salmonellosis in children.[15] In the first report, granulomatous osteomyelitis in a bearded dragon was associated with atypical mycobacteria.[13] The bearded dragon presented for a swollen stifle. A diagnostic workup (elevated white blood cell count, cytology, culture) confirmed that the animal had mycobacteriosis. Although the species of organism was not confirmed, it was presumed to be *M chelonae*. The owner of the animal wanted to pursue the case, so the leg was amputated and the bearded dragon treated with amikacin and erythromycin, which were both found to be effective against the mycobacterial isolate on sensitivity testing. The animal was lost to follow-up for 15 months, at which time it returned and presented for a large oral mass. The oral mass was confirmed to be a granuloma with acid-fast bacteria. Unfortunately, the animal died within 48 hours of re-presentation. In the second case, *M marinum* was the organism isolated from the bearded dragon.[14] The animal presented for anorexia and lethargy, common presentations for reptiles, along with joint swelling. Diagnostic tests revealed a significant elevation in the white blood cell count, similar to the first bearded dragon case, and miliary changes in the lungs. Joint aspirates revealed an inflammatory response along with acid-fast bacteria. A final diagnosis of mycobacteriosis (*M marinum*) was made using culture and polymerase chain reaction (PCR) analysis. The authors found it interesting that the species isolated from the bearded dragon is commonly associated with aquatic species, and after further questioning of the owner found that the animal had been fed dead guppies (*Poecilia* sp). This case demonstrated that certain practices could increase the likelihood of exposing an animal to a disease that it might not normally encounter. Also, although bearded dragons are ectotherms capable of obtaining basking body temperatures higher than those of endothermic vertebrates, and that *M marinum* is typically associated with aquatic poikilotherms with lower body temperatures (eg, fish and amphibians), the authors suspected that low environmental temperatures provided to the bearded dragon contributed to the infection. This should help further reinforce the importance of husbandry as it relates to the development of disease in reptiles.

MYCOBACTERIAL INFECTIONS IN SNAKES

Mycobacteriosis in snakes is a rare finding, with five reports documented since the late 1920s (see **Table 1**).[16–20] It is likely that mycobacteriosis is more common, but goes undiagnosed because complete necropsies are not performed.

There have been three reports of mycobacteriosis in boa constrictors (*Boa constrictor*), and the distribution of clinical disease was similar in all three cases even though the isolates were different in the two in which they were confirmed. In the first case, the snake was found to have systemic mycobacteriosis.[17] Lesions were found on the skin, in the oral cavity (stomatitis), and in the respiratory tract. *M thamnopheos* was isolated from the lesions in this snake. In the second report, *M chelonei* was isolated from the boa constrictor.[18] The animal presented with stomatitis and subcutaneous granulomas located over the dorsum. The pathogen was isolated from these sites as well as from the liver and lungs. The final boa case was found to have a *Mycobacterium* sp associated with an infectious stomatitis.[19] It is interesting that these animals had stomatitis, often generically called "mouth rot" by herpetoculturists.

This is a common presentation for snakes with focal or systemic disease, and these cases should reinforce the importance of performing diagnostic tests on an ill reptile, versus solely providing empirical treatment with antimicrobials.

The single report in a python was associated with a dual infection, M haemophilum and M marinum, in a royal or ball python (Python regius).[20] The affected snake was presented with a chronic history (18 months) of respiratory disease. Diagnosis was made by pursuing endoscopic examination of the lower respiratory tract, where diffuse, granulomatous disease was found. Histopathology was consistent with a pyogranulomatous inflammation, and acid-fast bacteria were found throughout the lesions. PCR testing and DNA sequencing were used to confirm the presence of the two mycobacteria. The snake was euthanized after diagnosis. The findings in this snake, as with the boa constrictors, should remind veterinarians of the importance of pursuing diagnostic testing in reptile cases. Although mycobacteriosis is uncommon in reptiles, respiratory disease is common.

MYCOBACTERIAL INFECTIONS IN CHELONIANS

Reports of mycobacteriosis in reptiles appear to be most common in chelonians (see **Table 1**).[12,21–24] This should not, however, come as a surprise because many of these cases are associated with an aquatic environment, where Mycobacterium spp are known to be ubiquitous. Having said that, there is at least one case report in a terrestrial species.[23] Therefore, veterinarians working with these animals should not exclude mycobacteriosis as a rule-out in tortoises that are presented with clinical signs consistent with this disease. Another important aspect of the epidemiology of the disease in chelonians is that, in the majority of cases, affected animals are either wild animals being brought into captivity[23,25] or free-ranging wild animals being rehabilitated in captivity.[12,26] Affected animals can develop a variety of clinical signs and pathology.

The majority of the mycobacteriosis cases in chelonians are described in sea turtles. Actually, the first report of mycobacteriosis in a turtle was in a sea turtle in 1903.[27] Since that time, a number of cases in different species of sea turtles have been reported.[24,26,28–30] In most cases, the sea turtle was presented for chronic disease and granulomatous lesions are found postmortem.[26,28] Although the disease is often associated with the lungs and viscera (liver, spleen, kidneys),[24,26,28] it has also been found to be associated with bone and joint tissues.[26] The findings in sea turtles suggest that the disease is spread hematogenously, so it is possible that the bacteria could end up in a variety of tissues. However, it is generally thought that the Mycobacterium spp gain systemic access through cutaneous routes, so protecting cutaneous lesions during the rehabilitation process may limit a sea turtle's exposure to these pathogens. This is especially important in animals undergoing rehabilitation because they tend to be considered immunocompromised and more susceptible to opportunistic infections.

Because Mycobacterium spp are capable of thriving in a variety of environmental conditions, it should come as no surprise that these pathogens are also found in freshwater chelonians. Several freshwater species of chelonians have been found to have mycobacteriosis. A wild caught side-necked turtle (Phrynops hilari) brought into captivity was found to become emaciated over a short period of time.[24] Other than cutaneous lesions that developed 5 months before death, the animal had no other clinical signs leading up to its death. At necropsy, granulomas were found in the liver and spleen. Acid-fast bacteria consistent with Mycobacteria sp were found in both organs and the cutaneous lesions. The authors suspected that the Mycobacterium was M chelonei, although no diagnostic tests were performed to confirm this.

Additional case reports in freshwater chelonians are similar in that they start with cutaneous lesions and then become chronic in nature with systemic granulomatous disease[22,24]; however, there are also exceptions. In at least one case, a spiny softshell turtle (*Apalone spinifera spinifera*) was presented for acute mycobacteriosis that was characterized by bacterial emboli with a disseminated intravascular coagulopathy.[12] This particular animal did not have any overt granulomatous disease, and the case should be a reminder that mycobacteriosis may not always present with a typical clinical picture of a chronic debilitating disease.

Although most reports of mycobacteriosis in chelonians are in aquatic species, mycobacteriosis has also been reported in a terrestrial chelonian. A box turtle (*Terrapene carolina carolina*) was presented for a soft tissue mass dorsal and to the right of its tail that eventually progressed to carapacial lesions.[23] Culture of the lesions eventually confirmed the presence of *M terrae*; however, time to isolation on culture was greater than 50 days. Although the animal showed some response to supportive care and antibiotic therapy, the disease eventually could not be controlled and euthanasia was elected. At postmortem the disease was found to be more than focal, with granulomas also noted in the liver, kidneys, spleen, and lungs. This isolation of *M terrae* in this case is interesting because it is relatively uncommon in vertebrates, and this case represented the first documented case in a reptile. The concern with this organism is that it is potentially zoonotic, and again reinforces the potential risk associated with working with these animals. The lesions noted were similar to those many clinicians see on first examination of a chelonian, and further reinforce the potential for misclassifying the true risk of mycobacteriosis in reptiles when thorough diagnostic workups are not performed.

REPTILES AS MODELS OF MYCOBACTERIAL INFECTION

For a period of time there was a strong interest in evaluating the potential role of reptiles in the epidemiology of *Mycobacterium* spp important to humans. It was thought that the reptiles could serve as animal models to evaluate diagnostic tests and potential therapies for humans. While these studies were being done, they also provided some insight into the role of reptiles in the epidemiology of these pathogens.

The role of snakes in the epidemiology of *M leprae* was evaluated.[31] Juvenile yellow rat snakes (*Elaphe quadrivitta*) were injected intramuscularly with a human isolate of *M leprae* (see **Table 1**). The isolate was either injected directly or after being heat treated. Snakes injected with a non-heat- treated form of the pathogen were found to become emaciated and experience significant weight loss; these snakes died within 11 to 13 weeks of treatment. The snakes given the heat-treated isolate survived but were euthanized at 5 months. The study showed that *M leprae* can infect snakes, and that snakes could transmit the organism between each other. The results suggest that snakes could harbor additional species of mycobacteria that are pathogenic to humans, and that body temperature did not limit the growth of this organism in the snakes.

Shortly after the snake study, additional studies were performed to evaluate the role of lizards in the epidemiology of another species of mycobacteria.[32,33] Green anoles (*Anolis carolinensis*) inoculated subcutaneously with viable *M ulcerans* were found to develop slowly progressive lesions at the site of inoculation (see **Table 1**).[32] Three different inflammatory responses were noted in the anoles. The most common was a diffuse, granulomatous response with intracellular acid-fast bacteria. The next most common response was a diffuse necrotizing granulomatous response with extracellular acid-fast bacteria. A focal encapsulated granuloma was found in only one lizard. A follow-up study evaluated the potential infectivity of *M ulcerans* in green anoles after oral inoculation of the bacteria via a stomach tube.[33] Inoculated anoles were found to actively shed the bacteria for up to 11 days after inoculation. Follow-up histopathology on the lizards showed that the organism had a predilection for the liver, with *M ulcerans* being isolated from the livers of 15% (3/20) of the lizards. Acid-fast bacteria were identified in the mucosa of the intrahepatic bile ducts in 66% (2/3) of the lizards in which the organism was found. The findings of the study reinforced that this species of lizard could serve as a reservoir or carrier of *M ulcerans*, leaving the door open to the fact that other reptiles may also serve a similar role in the epidemiology of this, and potentially other, mycobacteria. The findings also suggest that reptiles may be able to develop some form of resistance to these bacteria, reinforcing why the prevalence is low. Finally, it is also important to note that this study was performed before PCR testing became available, and that results may have been different (higher prevalence) had a more sensitive test been possible.

Because of the historic concerns of mycobacteriosis in humans, infection studies similar to that described in snakes have also been performed in turtles.[31] *Kinosternon leukostonum* were inoculated intracoelomically with *M leprae* and *M lepraemurium* to determine if these pathogens were infective to the turtles (see **Table 1**).[34] The primary interest of the researchers was similar to that defined by the individuals studying the snakes: to create a new model for *M leprae* infectivity to study diagnostics and treatments for humans. In the case of the turtles, the *M leprae* did not appear to infect the turtles, while *M lepraemurium* did cause a mild inflammatory response. This was in contrast to what was seen with the rat snakes.[31,34] The results do suggest that reptiles could potentially play a role in the epidemiology of the disease, but to what extent is unknown.

DIAGNOSING MYCOBACTERIAL INFECTIONS IN REPTILES

Histopathology is routinely used to diagnose mycobacteriosis in reptiles. Reptiles with mycobacteriosis tend to develop granulomatous lesions that are evident on hematoxylin–eosin stains. In many cases, these lesions are characterized by multi-nucleated giant cells.[5] Acid-fast stains, such as the Ziehl-Neelsen method and Fite's method, are commonly used to evaluate these granulomatous lesions further and look specifically for acid-fast bacteria such as mycobacteria. Unfortunately, the sensitivity of these stains can be low. In at least one study, a fluorescent method using auramine–phenol stain was found to be more sensitive than the fuchsin stains at diagnosing tuberculosis in humans.[35] When reviewing histopathology using these methods it is important to consider the potential for misclassification.

Historically, culture was used to confirm the presence of mycobacteria in reptiles. However, this method has lost favor with a number of diagnostic laboratories because of the special medias required for different *Mycobacteria* spp and the long culture (generation) times for these organisms. Fortunately, with the advent of PCR, it has become easier to achieve a final diagnosis for patients with mycobacteriosis. There are a number of primers available for characterizing mycobacteria. Primers for the 16S ribosomal RNA gene are commonly used in diagnostic laboratories in the United States. Recently, PCR was used to diagnose *M szulgai* in a *C johnstoni* and a *C crocodilus fuscus*.[2,5] The *hsp65* gene was targeted using a nested PCR. This gene encodes a 65-kDa heat shock protein. This same primer was used to perform a retrospective study to estimate the prevalence of mycobacteriosis in pathologic specimens from a collection in Switzerland.[36] It is important to evaluate the PCR methods used for assessing mycobacteria in a reptile, as there can be some variability in the sensitivity and specificity of the assay based on the type of sample, species, and primers used.

PREVALENCE OF MYCOBACTERIAL INFECTIONS IN REPTILES

Many of the case reports described in this review article suggest that mycobacteriosis is relatively uncommon in reptiles. However, as mentioned previously, it is possible that many cases go undiagnosed because of a lack of follow-through on cases by clinicians or pathologists. This may occur because of the financial constraints of an owner (eg, no necropsy performed) or limited experience and thus limited diagnostic capacity of the clinician or pathologist. To understand better the epidemiology of mycobacteriosis in reptiles, it is important to perform population-based studies to estimate the prevalence of this disease in reptiles. To date, a single cross-sectional study has been performed to estimate the prevalence of mycobacteria in reptiles.[36] The study utilized archived formalin-fixed tissue samples that had been characterized as having granulomatous inflammation. A total of 90 samples collected over a 10-year period were used. The samples were evaluated using Ziehl-Neelsen acid-fast stains and PCR (*hsp65* gene). A total of 14 (15.6%) samples were positive on the Ziehl-Neelsen stains, while 23 (25.6%) samples were PCR positive. The positive samples were associated with a variety of tissues, including the gastrointestinal, respiratory, and genitourinary tracts; heart; spleen; and central nervous system. The results of the study reinforce the importance of using sensitive testing methods for characterizing the mycobacteria status of a reptile, with PCR being more sensitive than either histopathology or acid-fast stains alone. The study also suggests that mycobacteriosis may not be an uncommon disease in reptiles, especially those found to have granulomatous disease. Veterinarians should consider this when working with reptiles found to have granulomatous disease.

ZOONOTIC POTENTIAL

It is worth mentioning that the majority of *Mycobacterium* spp isolated from reptiles are classified as atypical forms (eg, *M chelonae*). Many of these bacteria belong to the Runyon Group IV and are characterized as being resistant to antibiotics. These forms are not typically found in humans, but there are certainly case reports of disease in humans with these mycobacteria.[37] Therefore, it is important that veterinarians educate their staff and clients regarding the potential zoonotic threat of mycobacteriosis in reptiles. Children and individuals with compromised immune systems should take special precautions and avoid contact to minimize any potential risk of exposure. Currently, there are no proven or approved treatments for mycobacteriosis in reptiles, and because of the zoonotic potential of these bacteria, none are recommended at this time.

SUMMARY

Mycobacteriosis is an important disease worldwide. Although commonly associated with higher vertebrates, including humans, this disease has been reported in only a handful of reptile cases. The limited number of reports in reptiles may be associated with a low true prevalence of disease; however, it is also possible that cases go undiagnosed because of limited follow-through by veterinary clinicians and pathologists. When present, this disease appears to present as a chronic debilitating disease, although at least one example of an acute presentation exists. Mycobacteriosis appears to be most common in aquatic reptiles, especially those in production systems such as crocodilians. The potential zoonotic status of these organisms is sound reason for veterinarians to educate their clients regarding the need for case follow-up to rule in or rule out the potential presence of these pathogens in pet reptiles and best handling practices to minimize their exposure.

REFERENCES

1. Huchzermeyer FW. Crocodile biology, husbandry, and diseases. Wallingford (UK): CABI; 2003.
2. Slany M, Knotek Z, Skoric M, et al. Systemic mixed infection in a brown caiman (*Caiman crocodilus fuscus*) caused by *Mycobacterium szulgai* and *M. chelonae*: a case report. Vet Med 2010;55(2):91–6.
3. Nevarez J. Crocodilian differential diagnosis. In: Mader DR, editor. Reptile medicine and surgery. 2nd edition. St. Louis (MO): Saunders/Elsevier; 2005. p. 705–14.
4. Youngprapakorn P, Ousavaplanchai L, Kanchanapangka S. A color atlas of diseases of the crocodile. Bangkok (Thailand): Style Creative; 1994. p. 95.
5. Roh YS, Park H, Cho A, et al. Granulamotous pneumonia in a captive freshwater crocodile (*Crocodylus johnstoni*) caused by *Mycobacterium szulgai*. J Zoo Wildl Med 2010;41(93):550–4.
6. Buenviaje GN, Ladds PW, Martin Y. Pathology of skin diseases in reptiles. Aust Vet J 1998;76(5):357–63.
7. Ariel E, Ladds PW, Roberts BL. Mycobacteriosis in young freshwater crocodiles (*Crocodylus johnstoni*). Aust Vet J 1997;75(11):831–3.
8. Huchzermeyer FW. Public health risks of ostrich and crocodile meat. Rev Sci Tech 1997;16(20:599–604.
9. Maloney JM, Gregg CR, Stephens DS, et al. Infections caused by *Mycobacterium szulgai* in humans. Rev Infect Dis 1987;9(6):1120–6.
10. Friend SCE, Russell EG. *Mycobacterium intracellulare* infection in a water monitor. J Wildl Dis 1979;15:229–33.
11. Morales P, Dunker F. Fish tuberculosis, *Mycobacterium marinum*, in a group of Egyptian spiny tailed lizards, *Uromastyx aegypticus*. J Herp Med Surg 2001;11: 27–30.
12. Murray M, Waliszewski NT, Garnerr MM, et al. Sepsis and disseminated intravascular coagulation in an eastern spiny softshell turtle (*Apalone spinifera spinifera*) with acute mycobacteriosis. J Zoo Wildl Med 2009;40(3):572–5.
13. Kramer MH. Granulomatous osteomyelitis associated with atypical mycobacteria in a bearded dragon (*Pogona vitticeps*). Vet Clin North Am Exot Anim Pract 2006;9(3): 563–8.
14. Girling SJ, Fraser MA. Systemic mycobacteriosis in an inland bearded dragon (*Pogona vitticeps*). Vet Rec 2007;160:526–8.
15. Mitchell MA. Zoonotic diseases associated with reptiles and amphibians: an update. Vet Clin North Am Exot Anim Pract 2011;14(3):439–56.
16. Aronson JD. Spontaneous tuberculosis in snakes. J Infect Dis 1929;44:215–23.
17. Kiel M. Reptilian tuberculosis in a boa constrictor. J Zoo Wildl Anim Med 1977;8:9–11.
18. Quesenberry KE, Jacobson ER, Allen JL, et al. Ulcerative stomatitis and subcutaneous granulomas caused by *Mycobacterium chelonei* in a boa constrictor. J Am Vet Med Assoc 1986; 189(9):1131–2.
19. Olsen GH, Hodgin C, Pechman R. Infectious stomatitis associated with *Mycobacterium* sp. in a boa constrictor. Comp Anim Pract 1987;47-49.
20. Hernandez-Divers SJ, Shearer D. Pulmonary mycobacteriosis caused by *Mycobacteriumm haemophilum* and *M. marinum* in a royal python. J Am Vet Med Assoc 2002;220(11):1661–3.
21. Doyle RE, Moreland AF. Diseases of turtles. Lab Anim Dig 1968;4:3–6.
22. Oros J, Acosta B, Gaskin JM, et al. *Mycobacterium kansasii* in a Chinese soft-shelled turtle (*Pelodiscus sinensis*). Vet Rec 2003;152:474–6.

23. Noyes H, Bronson E, Deem S, et al. Systemic *Mycobacterium terrae* infection in an Eastern box turtle, *Terrapene carolina carolina*. J Herp Med Surg 2007;17(3):100–2.

24. Rhodin AGJ, Anver MR. Mycobacteriosis in turtles: cutaneous and hepatosplenic involvement in a *Phrynops hilari*. J Wildl Dis 1977;13:180–3.

25. Schildiger BJ, Weub R, Frank H, et al. Mycobacteriosis in Australian snake neck turtles (*Chelodina longicollis*). In: Proceedings of the 4th International Colloquium on Pathology and Medicine of Reptiles and Amphibians. Bad Nauheim (Germany), September 27–29, 1991.

26. Greer LL, Strandberg JD, Whitaker BR. *Mycobacterium chelonae* osteoarthritis in a Kemp's ridley sea turtle (*Lepidochelys kempii*). J Wildl Dis 2003;39(3):736–41.

27. Friedmann FF. Spontane Lungentuberkulose bei Schildkroten und die Stellung des Tuberkelbazillus im System. Zeitschr Tuberk 1903;4:439–57.

28. Brock JA, Nakamura RM, Miyahara AY, et al. Tuberculosis in Pacific green turtles, *Chelonia mydas*. Trans Am Fish Soc 1976;105:564–6.

29. Keymer IF. Diseases of chelonians: 1) Necropsy survey of tortoises. Vet Rec 1978; 103:548–52.

30. Glazebrook JS, Campbell RSF. A survey of diseases of marine turtles in northern Australia. I. Farmed turtles. Dis Aquat Organ 1990;9:83–95.

31. Kwapinski JB, Kwapinski EH, McClung NM. The growth of *Mycobacterium leprae* in snakes. Can J Microbiol 1974;20(3):420–2.

32. Marcus LC, Stottmeier KD, Morrow RH. Experimental infection of anole lizards (*Anolis carolinensis*) with *Mycobacterium ulcerans* by the subcutaneous route. Am J Trop Med Hyg 1975;24(4):649–55.

33. Marcus LC, Stottmeier KD, Morrow RH. Experimental alimentary infection of anole lizards (*Anolis carolinensis*) with *Mycobacterium ulcerans*. Am J Trop Med Hyg 1976;25(4):630–2.

34. Rojas-Espinosa O, Quesada-Pascual F, Estrada-Parra S, et al. An attempt to infect turtles (*Kinosternon leucostonum*) with *Mycobacterium leprae* and *M. lepraemurium*. Dev Comp Immunol 1985;9(1):147–50.

35. Greenwood N, Fox H. A comparison of methods for staining tubercle bacilli in histologic sections. J Clin Pathol 1973;26:253–7.

36. Soldati G, Lu ZH, Vaughn L, et al. Detection of mycobacteria and chlamydiae in granulomatous inflammation of reptiles: a retrospective study. Vet Pathol 2004;41: 388–97.

37. Brown TH. The rapidly growing mycobacteria-*Mycobacteria fortuitum* and *Mycobacterium chelonei*. Infect Control 1985;6(7):283–8.

Amphibian Mycobacteriosis

Filipe Martinho, DVM[a], J. Jill Heatley, DVM, MS, Dipl ABVP (Avian), Dipl ACZM[b],*

KEYWORDS

- Amphibian • *Mycobacterium* • Anuran • Caudate
- Zoonosis • Mycobacteria • Celomic effusion

Amphibians are commonly kept in laboratory and zoological facilities and are becoming more frequent as pets. A variety of captive bred species are now available, including brightly colored dart frogs, large Pac-man frogs, and small aquatic species. As care, feeding, and other husbandry techniques continue to improve, these animals will likely become more popular as pets. However, many amphibian species are declining in the wild owing to a variety of infectious and noninfectious diseases. The true prevalence of mycobacteriosis in wild amphibian species remains unknown; most reports of amphibian mycobacteriosis stem from captive frog colonies. However, although diagnostics continue to improve, effective cure of this devastating disease is still elusive. This article reviews the current state of knowledge of mycobacteriosis in amphibian species, including pathogenesis, clinical signs, appropriate diagnostics, treatment options, and zoonotic potential and prevention. It is hoped this review will provide clinical veterinarians and scientists the tools they need to provide better care for amphibian species suffering mycobacteriosis, as well as serve to stimulate additional research into amphibians affected by mycobacterosis.

SPECIES OF *MYCOBACTERIUM* DETECTED IN AMPHIBIANS

A number of *Mycobacterium* species have been detected and described in amphibians (**Table 1**). Captive amphibians in collections and laboratory models and free-living animals have been affected, including caecilians, anurans, and caudates. Generally, mycobacteriosis has been reported in adult animals, after metamorphosis. The majority of mycobacterial infections in amphibians have been reported in African clawed frogs (*Xenopus* sp),[1–5] probably because this species is used in biomedical research and there are large captive populations worldwide, receiving more veterinary care than other amphibian species. There also have been some reports of infection in

Disclosure: The authors have nothing to disclose.

[a] Faculdade de Medicina Veterinária, Universidade Lusófona de Humanidades e Tecnologias, Lisbon, Portugal

[b] Department of Small Animal Clinical Sciences, Zoological Medicine Service, College of Veterinary Medicine and Biomedical Sciences, Texas A&M University, College Station, TX 77843-4474, USA

* Corresponding author.

E-mail address: JHeatley@cvm.tamu.edu

Table 1
Amphibian mycobacteriosis

Mycobacterial Species	Amphibian Species Affected	Infection Type	References
M marinum	Silurana [Xenopus] tropicalis (African clawed frog)	Natural	Taylor et al[21]
	Xenopus laevis (South African clawed frog)	Natural	Cannon et al[25]
	Rana pipiens (Northern leopard frog)	Experimental	Ramakrishnan et al[10]
	Hoplobatrachus [Rana] tigrina (Indus Valley bullfrog)	Experimental	Pranwichien et al[29]
	Rana catesbeiana (American bullfrog)	Natural	Ferreira et al,[6] Maslow et al,[7] Moraes[8]
	Pyxicephalus adspersus (African bullfrog)	Natural	Pizzi & Miller[13]
	Acris sp (cricket frogs)	Experimental	Clark & Shepard[16]
	Chaunus [Bufo] spinolosus, B cognatus, B woodhousii (Woodhouses's toad)	Natural	Shiveley et al[14]
M chelonei	Xenopus laevis	Natural	Green et al[3]
	Bufo marinus, Chaunus [Bufo] granulosus	Natural	Mok & Carvalho[12]
M fortuitum	Leptodactylus pentadactylus (smoky jungle frog)	Natural	Darzins[30]
M xenopi	Xenopus laevis	Natural	Taylor et al[21]
M avium intracellulare complex	Xenopus tropicalis	Natural	Chai et al[1]
M liflandii	Xenopus tropicalis	Natural	Suykerbuyk et al[4]
	Xenopus laevis	Natural	Godfrey et al[2]
	Leptodactylus pentadactylus	Natural	Rowlatt & Roe[22]
M szulgai	Xenopus tropicalis	Natural	Chai et al[1]
M gordonae	Xenopus tropicalis, Xenopus laevis	Natural	Kirsch,[24] Sánchez-Morgado et al[28]
Mycobacterium sp unknown	Cynops [Triturus] pyrrhogaster (Japanese fire belly newt)	Natural	Shiveley et al[14]
M ulcerans	Xenopus laevis	Natural	Godfrey et al,[2] Mve-Obiang et al,[18] Portaels et al[26]

bullfrogs (*Rana catesbeiana*)[6–9] and leopard frogs (*Rana pipiens*),[10] which are either commercially raised in frog farms or are occasionally used in biomedical research, but very few in pet or zoo amphibians or wild populations or individuals.[11–14] *M marinum* has been the most frequently isolated mycobacterium in amphibians but other species, which commonly infect other poikilothermic animals, have also been detected, such as *M chelonae*. Some species of mycobacteria have been isolated only from amphibians, such as *M liflandi*. However, regarding mycobacterial species, clinicians should understand that as genetic diagnostic techniques have progressed, previous diagnoses of mycobacterial species may not reflect the current classification; moreover, some may also be consistent with newer species more recently described.

PATHOGENESIS

Mycobacteria appear to be transmitted to amphibians through direct contact between infected individuals, contaminated water, and fomites. Nevertheless, other ways of transmission should not be excluded. The infective dose is very low, about 23 bacteria per individual.[13] Some Mycobacteria species, such as *M marinum* and *M ulcerans*, appear to be ubiquitous in aquatic environments, at least in some parts of the world.

Usually, in immunocompetent individuals, mycobacteria induce a chronic subclinical infection with few, if any, clinical signs. In stressed and immunodepressed amphibians, such as those housed in crowded environments or with incorrect temperature or water parameters, the course of infection is much more severe, leading to systemic and acute disease.[6,10,15,16]

As in tuberculosis and other mycobacterioses, the infection in amphibians is characterized by chronic inflammation and the presence of granulomatous lesions. These granulomas are the amphibian's attempt to contain the bacteria. These granulomas are composed of variable numbers of lymphocytes, macrophages, epithelioid cells, fibroblasts, and sometimes melanocytes, enclosing a necrotic or sometimes caseous center containing mycobacteria.[5,15,17]

M liflandi is a unique mycobacteria that infects amphibians and produces a toxin, Mycolactone E, that has direct cytopathic effects, leading to fibroblast apoptosis and an increased inflammatory response.[4,18]

CLINICAL SIGNS AND SYNDROMES OF AMPHIBIANS AFFECTED BY MYCOBACTERIOSIS

Mycobacteriosis can present as a chronic or subclinical infection with few or no signs or as acute disease with a high mortality rate. In symptomatic amphibians, clinical signs are often vague and nonpathognomonic and one can only suspect mycobacteriosis based on clinical examination. Clinical signs of mycobacteriosis vary based on the species of mycobacteria, the species of amphibian, and environmental conditions. It is of extreme clinical importance to note that a large percentage of individuals in an infected group may lack clinical signs.[6] Mycobacteriosis should be suspected in any amphibian with nonspecific signs of illness, weight loss, lethargy, anorexia, bloating, or ulcerative or nodular dermatitis. Subcutaneous edema, celomic effusion, bloating, and abnormal buoyancy have been described and may be more apparent in aquatic species, such as *Xenopus* sp.[2,4,5,9,19] Dermatologic lesions are common and include areas of skin hyperemia, petechiae, ulcers, and nodules.[2,4–6,14,19–21] These lesions can be diffuse or localized. In acute disease, the only sign may be sudden death, and infected animals are more prone to opportunistic or secondary infections.[2,8,19] Infections localized to the eye have also been described.[22]

Clinical signs may vary based on the mycobacterial species involved as follows: *M marinum* can cause reluctance to dive, celomic effusion, loss of dive reflex, and abdominal distension as well as skin lesions on the head and extremities.[6,23] *M marinum* causes both long-term subclinical infection and acute disease. Chronic granulomatous nonlethal disease often occurs in immunocompetent frogs whereas frogs that are immunosuppressed suffer acute disease resulting in death.[22] *M gordonae* has caused granulomatous lesions of the toe tips of *Xenopus laevis*.[24] *M liflandii* has caused acute celomic distension, accumulation of serosanguinous fluid in the subcutaneous space or body cavity, and fatality in frogs.[2,4] *M szulgai* infection has been associated with lethargy, weight loss, and emaciation in amphibians.[1] *M chelonae* has caused chronic weight loss and ulcerative skin lesions.[3] An *M ulcerans*-like organism has caused lethargy, excess buoyancy, celomic effusion, cutaneous ulcers, ulcerative and granulomatous dermatitis, celomitis, and septicemia in amphibians.[5] *Mycobacterium* spp have also been causative of glomerulonephritis and anasarca, hydrocelom, and swelling and ecchymoses of the mandible.[25,26]

DIAGNOSIS

Methods for diagnosis of mycobacterial disease in amphibians are based on discovery and correct identification of the infective organism. Methods include fluid analysis, biopsy accompanied by cytologic analysis, histopathology, and culture and traditional biochemical or polymerase chain reaction (PCR) gene probe identification. Antemortem diagnosis is possible but postmortem diagnosis is more commonly documented in amphibians.

Dead and euthanized individuals should be subject to thorough necropsy and complete investigation. Infected animals usually have a variable number of small to large granulomas affecting the skin and almost any internal organ but especially the liver.[2,5,8,9,14,22] Other lesions such as pulmonary congestion,[14] celomitis, and ascites have also been described[2,4,5,7,9] and should be targeted for etiologic diagnosis and confirmation of mycobacteriosis.

Ziehl-Nielsen stain can be used for imprints of skin ulcers, cytologic preparations from lesion or celomic aspirates, or organ imprints. Mycobacteria stain as red to pink filamentous rods against a blue/green background.

Mycobacterium spp can be cultured and isolated in a number of mediums. Because most of the *Mycobacterium* spp that infect amphibians grow at relatively low temperatures, the incubation temperature should be about 23°C to 30° C. Mycobacteria are fastidious and slow-growing bacteria, so it usually takes a few weeks to obtain a positive culture result.[2,6,7,12,16,20]

In recent years, it has been possible to detect and identify *Mycobacterium* spp by molecular methods and a number of PCR-based techniques, increasing specificity and sensitivity and decreasing waiting time for results. Species identification and characterization can be made with restriction fragment length polymorphism (RFLP) analysis or other molecular techniques or with high-performance liquid chromatography (HPLC).[2–4,6,7] *Mycobacterium* spp should be differentiated from other infectious agents such as ranavirus, *Batrachochytrium dendrobatidis*, *Chlamydophila* spp, *Aeromonas hydrophila*, and unspecific bacteria or fungi, as well as cutaneous neoplasms such as lymphosarcoma or histiocytoma. In bloated individuals, mycobacteriosis should be differentiated from other systemic infections; neoplasia; internal parasites; liver, renal, or heart failure; and, in adult females, reproductive tract disorders.[4,20]

TREATMENT

Although occasionally some treatment approaches have been attempted, such as amputation of infected distal parts[13] or administration of azithromycin or clarithromycin,[3] the risk of systemic disease or recurrence of infection is very high. Some studies suggest that the *Mycobacterium* spp that infect amphibians are multiresistant to drugs such as isoniazid, ethambutol, rifampin, clarithromycin, and ethionamide.[4] Effective treatments for mycobacteriosis in amphibians remain unreported. Therefore, at this time, and due to zoonotic potential, culling or euthanasia of affected amphibians and appropriate postmortem examination and diagnosis, precise identification of the mycobacteria involved, and disinfection are recommended in most cases.[20]

The incidence of mycobacteriosis can be decreased by providing optimal husbandry for each species, reducing stress and overpopulation, ensuring good hygiene, removing abrasive objects or substrates from the tank, and by prompt diagnosis and isolation of suspected cases. Mycobacteria are resistant to ultraviolet radiation, and some disinfectants such as glutaraldehyde but sensitive to 200 ppm bleach solutions and 70% ethanol. For prevention, new animals should be quarantined and properly examined before introducing to established tanks.[2,3,9,27]

ZOONOTIC CONSIDERATIONS

There are no known reports in the literature of direct transmission of mycobacteria from amphibians to humans. Human infection seems more likely to occur when water contaminated with bacteria comes in contact with skin wounds or abrasions. Trauma at the site of skin contamination and direct contact are important factors in most of these infections. Therefore, all infected amphibians should be handled while wearing nonpowdered and moist latex gloves, not only to reduce the risk of pathogen transmission but also to minimize the disruption of the amphibian skin mucous layer.

Although rare, infection in humans with many of these species of *Mycobacterium* described has been reported, causing ulcerative or nodular dermatitis, especially on the extremities. The species more commonly isolated in humans are *M marinum*, which causes a syndrome referred as aquarium tank granuloma[6,17] and *M ulcerans*, the causative agent of Buruli ulcer.[5,18] *M gordonae* is also an occasional human pathogen causing cutaneous infections and nodular granulomatous skin lesions.[28] *M chelonae* have also been isolated in human patients with chronic skin abscesses and nonhealing erosive skin ulcers.[3]

M marinum causes occasional granulomatous lesions localized in the skin, typically after minor trauma to the hands. This disease is common in aquarium keepers and can infrequently spread to tendon sheaths or joints. Dissemination is rare and occurrence is limited to immunosuppressed patients. Buruli ulcer is the third most common mycobacterial disease of humans and can cause serious deformities and disabilities. This agent is associated with and proliferates in the mud and stagnant waters of tropical wetlands in Africa. Transmission involves direct contact with environmental contamination but also aerosols from water surfaces and with water-dwelling insects. Disease may vary from a localized nodule to widespread ulcerated or nonulcerated disease including osteomyelitis. The host range of experimental infection for *M ulcerans* includes amphibians; however, no natural infection has been observed.[26]

SUMMARY

Mycobacteriosis is a common disease of bacterial etiology in amphibians that causes chronic, sometimes lethal, disease. Multiple mycobacterial species have been found in a variety of amphibian species. The mycobacteria more frequently isolated in this group of animals, *Mycobacterium marinum, M fortuitum, M ulcerans, M chelonae*, and *M liflandi*, can cause ulcerative skin disease or generalized infection with multiple granuloma formation. Clinical signs are not pathognomonic for mycobacteriosis. Diagnosis is complex and best based on a combination of histopathologic, culture, and PCR diagnostics. Based on zoonotic concerns and a lack of response to treatment in previous cases, amphibians are seldom treated for mycobacteriosis. Quarantine, husbandry appropriate to the species, disinfection, and low numbers of animals per enclosure are appropriate preventative measures to avoid introduction and dissemination of mycobacteria to captive amphibians.

REFERENCES

1. Chai N, Deforges L, Sougakoff W, et al. *Mycobacterium szulgai* infection in a captive population of African clawed frogs (*Xenopus tropicalis*). J Zoo Wildlife Med 2006;37(1): 55–8.
2. Godfrey D, Williamson H, Silverman J, et al. Newly identified *Mycobacterium* species in a *Xenopus laevis* colony. Comp Med 2006;57(1):97–104.
3. Green SL, Lifland BD, Bouley DM, et al. Disease attributed to *Mycobacterium chelonae* in South African clawed frogs (*Xenopus laevis*). Comp Med 2000;50(6): 675–9.
4. Suykerbuyk P, Vleminkx K, Pasmans F, et al. *Mycobacterium liflandi* infection in European colony of *Silurana tropicalis*. Emerg Infect Dis 2007;13(5):743–6.
5. Trott KA, Stacy BA, Lifland BD, et al. Characterization of a *Mycobacterium ulcerans*-like infection in a colony of African tropical clawed frogs (*Xenopus laevis*). Comp Med 2004;54(3):309–17.
6. Ferreira R, Fonseca LS, Afonso AM, et al. A report of mycobacteriosis caused by *Mycobacterium marinum* in bullfrogs (*Rana catesbeiana*). Vet J 2006;171:177–80.
7. Maslow JN, Wallace R, Michaels M, et al. Outbreak of *Mycobacterium marinum* among captive snakes and bullfrogs. Zoo Biol 2002;21:233–41.
8. Moraes JRE, Martins ML, Souza VN, et al. Anatomopathological diagnosis of myco-bacteriosis in bullfrogs (*Rana catesbeiana* Shaw, 1802) from Brazilian commercial frog farms. ARS Veterinaria 1999;15(2):110–4.
9. Vannevel JY. Glomerulonephritis and anasarca in a colony of frogs. Vet Clin Exotic Anim Pract 2006;9:609–16.
10. Ramakrishnan L, Valdivia RH, McKerrow JH, et al. *Mycobacterium marinum* causes both long-term subclinical infection and acute disease in the leopard frog (*Rana pipiens*). Infect Immun 1997;65(2):767–73.
11. Mok WY, Carvalho CM, Barreto da silva MS. Host-parasite relationship between amazonian anurans and atypical mycobacteria (*Mycobacterium chelonae* and *M. fortuitum*). Biotropica 1987;19(3):274–7.
12. Mok WY, Carvalho CM. Occurrence and experimental infection of toads (*Bufo marinus* and *B. granulosus*) with *Mycobacterium chelonae* subsp. *abscessus*. J Med Microbiol 1984;18:327–33.
13. Pizzi R, Miller J. Amputation of a *Mycobacterium marinum*-infected hindlimb in an African bullfrog (*Pyxicephalus adspersus*). Vet Rec 2005;156(23):747–8.
14. Shively JN, Songer JG, Prchal S, et al. *Mycobacterium marinum* infection in bufo-nidae. J Wildlife Dis 1981;17(1):3–7.

15. Bouley DM, Ghori N, Mercer KL, et al. Dynamic nature of host-pathogen interactions in *Mycobacterium marinum* granulomas. Infect Immun 2001;69(12):7820–31.
16. Clark HF, Shepard CC. Effect of environmental temperatures on infection with *Mycobacterium marinum* (Balnei) on mice and a number of poikilothermic species. J Bacteriol 1963;86:1057–69.
17. Asfari M. Mycobacterium-induced infectious granuloma in *Xenopus*: histopathology and transmissibility. Cancer Res 1988;48:958–63.
18. Mve-Obiang A, Lee RE, Umstot ES, et al. A newly discovered mycobacterial pathogen isolated from laboratory colonies of *Xenopus* species with lethal infections produces a new form of mycolactone, the *Mycobacterium ulcerans* macrolide toxin. Infect Immun 2005; 73(6):3307–12.
19. Hill WA, Newman SJ, Craig L, et al. Diagnosis of *Aeromonas hydrophila*, *Mycobacterium* species and *Batrachochytrium dendrobatidis* in an African clawed frog (*Xenopus laevis*). J Am Assoc Lab Anim Sci 2010;49(2):215–20.
20. Densmore CL, Green DE. Diseases of amphibians. ILAR J 2007;48(3):235–54.
21. Taylor SK, Green DE, Wright KM, et al. Bacterial diseases. In: Wright KM, Whitaker BR, editors. Amphibian medicine and captive husbandry. Malabar (FL): Krieger Publishing; 2001. p. 159–80.
22. Rowlatt UF, Roe FJC. Generalized tuberculosis in a South American frog *Leptodactylus pentadactylus*. Pathol Vet 1966;3:451–60.
23. Tarigo J, Linder K, Neel J, et al. Reluctant to dive: coelomic effusion in a frog. Vet Clin Path 2006;35(3):341–4.
24. Kirsch P, Nusser P, Hotzel H, et al. [*Mycobacterium gordonae* as potential cause of granulomatous lesions of the toe tips in the South African clawed frog (*Xenopus laevis*)]. Berl Munch Tierarztl Wochenschr 2008;121(7–8):270–7.
25. Cannon CZ, Linder K, Brizuela BJ, et al. Marked swelling with coalescing ecchymoses of the lower mandible in a *Xenopus laevis* frog. Lab Anim [NY] 2006;35(5):19–22.
26. Portaels F, Chemlal K, Elsen P, et al. *Mycobacterium ulcerans* in wild animals. Rev Sci Tech 2001;20(1):252–64.
27. Pessier AP. An overview of amphibian skin disease. Semin Avian Exotic Pet 2002; 11(3):162–74.
28. Sánchez-Morgado JM, Gallagher A, Johnson LK. *Mycobacterium gordonae* infection in a colony of African clawed frogs (*Xenopus tropicalis*). Lab Anim 2009;43(3):300–3.
29. Pranwichien K, Somsiri T, Chinabut S. Comparative study of experimental mycobacteriosis between snakeheadfish (*Chana striata*) and frog (*Rana tigrina*). Asian Fish Sci 1999;12:351–6.
30. Darzins E. The epizootic of tuberculosis among the gias in Bahia. Acta Tubercul Scand 1952;26(1):70–174.

Mycobacterial Infection in the Ferret

Christal Pollock, DVM, Dipl. ABVP-Avian*

KEYWORDS

- Ferret • *Mycobacterium* • Lymphadenitis
- Bovine tuberculosis • New Zealand

Mycobacteriosis is an important disease in the feral ferret (*Mustela putorius furo*) of New Zealand.[1–6] Elsewhere in the world reports of tuberculosis in the ferret are sporadic.[7–11] Genus *Mycobacterium* consists of aerobic, non–spore-forming, gram-positive, nonmotile bacteria that characteristically feature a cell wall rich in mycolic acids and esters.[8] Species isolated most commonly from ferrets include *Mycobacterium bovis, M avium,* and other members of the *M avium* complex (MAC) and *M triplex.*[3,12] Other species identified in ferrets include *M celatum, M abscessus, M genavense, M microti, M fortuitum, M florentinum, M interjectum, M septicum,* and *M peregrinum,* as well as 3 unidentified species in New Zealand ferrets.[3,8–10,13–16]

INCIDENCE AND CLINICAL SIGNS

With the notable exception of New Zealand, reports of tuberculosis in the ferret are relatively uncommon.[9] Tuberculosis used to be reported somewhat frequently in European laboratory colonies; however, the incidence dropped considerably once the raw meat and unpasteurized milk fed to ferrets were replaced with formulated diets.[12,17]

Most accounts of tuberculosis in the ferret are in middle-aged to older animals. In a survey of ferrets with *M bovis* infection, none of 35 infected animals were under 4 months of age.[5] Each 6-month age increment was associated with a 2.8-fold increase in the risk of infectious disease.[5]

CASE REPORTS INVOLVING NON–*MYCOBACTERIUM BOVIS* INFECTION IN FERRETS
Disease Involving the Gastrointestinal Tract

Mycobacterial infections most commonly affect the gastrointestinal tract and/or liver in the ferret.[18] Reports of granulomatous enteritis and hepatitis have been attributed to *Mycobacterium avium* complex in privately owned and laboratory ferrets.[11,17,19] *M avium* subspp *paratuberculosis* infection was described in both feral and laboratory

The author has nothing to disclose.
Lafeber Company, 24981 North 1400 East Road, Cornell, IL 61319, USA
* 1500 Huntington Lane, Cleveland Heights, OH 44118.
E-mail address: christal7@mac.com

ferrets.[18,19] In all cases, severe granulomatous inflammation within the mesenteric lymph nodes, liver, spleen, and/or intestinal tract was present.[11] Clinical signs described included anorexia, debilitation, progressive weight loss, vomiting, chronic diarrhea, and/or evidence of maldigestion and malabsorption.[11,19]

Disease Involving the Respiratory Tract

Pulmonary infection caused by M avium complex, M celatum, and M abscessus has also been described in ferrets.[8,14,20] Underlying upper respiratory tract disease caused by influenza virus may have played a role in the development of M abscessus pneumonia.[8]

Splenitis

M celatum was the cause of splenitis in a 5-year-old male castrated pet ferret with progressive weight loss, pallor, and splenomegaly. Fine needle aspiration of the spleen revealed extramedullary hematopoiesis as well as marked macrophage-dominated inflammation associated with a low number of acid-fast bacilli.[10]

Disseminated Infection

There are also reports in the literature of disseminated or generalized mycobacteriosis in ferrets caused by M genavense, M celatum, M microti, and M avium complex.[7,9,13,15,16] M avium complex has been identified as a cause of otitis media/interna, dermatitis, and meningoencephalitis in the ferret.[7] Clinical signs vary with the site of infection but may include head tilt, circling, lethargy, and vomiting.[7]

Disseminated M genavense infection included prominent conjunctival lesions in two adult ferrets.[9] The first animal exhibited generalized peripheral lymphadenopathy and a proliferative lesion on the nictitating membrane (**Fig. 1**). The second ferret had conjunctival swelling, serous ocular discharge, and swelling of the subcutaneous tissues of the nasal planum.[9]

Disseminated M celatum infection caused tuberculous lesions in the trachea, lungs, stomach wall, liver, and lymph nodes of a 4-year-old male ferret. The ferret presented with a cough, depression, and a 6-month history of weight loss.[15]

There are also 2 reports of M microti isolation in the ferret.[13,16] Clinical details are available in only one report in which the ferret presented with a history of anorexia, weight loss, and malaise. At necropsy, a disseminated infection was identified with numerous acid-fast bacteria in all organ tissues.[16]

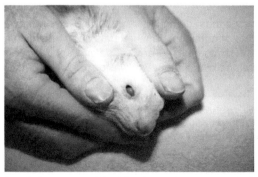

Fig. 1. Swelling of the nictitans caused by *Mycobacterium genavense* infection in an adult ferret (*Mustela putorius furo*). (*Courtesy of* Dr Richard Malik.)

The relationship between mycobacteriosis and a weakened immune system has been well established in human medicine.[21] Immunosuppression has also been theorized to play a role in tuberculous infections in the ferret.[9,22] Lymphosarcoma may have predisposed a 6-year-old male castrated ferret to *M avium* complex infection. Acid-fast organisms were widely disseminated with granulomatous inflammation found within the stomach, mesenteric lymph nodes, liver, kidneys, and lungs.[22]

MYCOBACTERIUM BOVIS INFECTION IN NEW ZEALAND
Bovine Tuberculosis in New Zealand

Bovine tuberculosis is an important infectious disease of domestic cattle and farmed deer herds in New Zealand.[2,17,23] The natural host of *M bovis* is cattle; however, this organism can infect a wide range of mammals.[24]

Like many developed nations, New Zealand began to practice standard test and slaughter methods in the mid-20th century in an effort to eradicate bovine tuberculosis.[2] By the late 1960s, it had become clear these tactics were not working.[2,24] The failure to eradicate bovine tuberculosis was attributed to the continual spread of *M bovis* from wildlife reservoir populations to livestock.[2,24,25] Transmission of tuberculosis from wildlife to livestock has been postulated to occur through pasture contamination as well as through direct investigation of dead or terminally ill animals behaving abnormally.[23,26] The Australian or common brushtail possum (*Trichosurus vulpecula*) is the principal wildlife reservoir of *M bovis* in New Zealand.[4,23,24,27,28]

Mycobacteriosis in Ferrets in New Zealand

New Zealand is believed to support the largest population of wild ferrets in the world.[2,17] Ferrets were originally released in the 1880s to control rabbit populations.[2,17,19]

Mycobacteriosis was first reported in feral ferrets in New Zealand in the early 1970s[4] but was not confirmed by culture until 1982.[24] Compared to other feral carnivores in New Zealand, like stoats (*Mustela erminea*) and domestic cats, only ferret populations have a high incidence of mycobacteriosis.[5,22,27,29] Surveys in endemic areas demonstrate prevalence up to 20% in some ferret populations.[23,24] Some authors have proposed the incidence of disease may be even higher due to the presence of subclinical disease.[4,23] Mycobacteriosis in the New Zealander ferret is most commonly caused by *M bovis*; however, *M avium* complex and *M triplex* are also frequently isolated.[3]

Epidemiology of Mycobacterium bovis Infection in Ferrets

A large proportion of lesions seen in ferrets with *M bovis* infection are found within the lymph nodes that drain the gastrointestinal tract. This suggests disease is transmitted to ferrets by ingestion of tuberculous prey or carrion such as dead possums or domestic animals discarded in offal pits.[2,5,6,27,30–32] Wild ferrets feed primarily on small mammals like rabbits but they also supplement their diet with a variety of other foods including carrion.[27] In areas in which *M bovis* infection is known to occur in ferret populations, a positive correlation has been demonstrated between possum numbers and the prevalence of *M bovis* infection in feral ferrets.[30,31]

Infected ferrets may spread *M bovis* in a variety of ways. Based on culture of various samples, the most common route of excretion is the ferret oral cavity.[5] *M bovis* has also been isolated from 4 of 64 tracheobronchial lavage samples (6 %), 10 of 63 fecal samples (16%), 2 of 29 urine samples (7%), and 1 of 8 mammary glands (12.5%).[5]

Horizontal transmission of *M bovis* is believed to occur within ferret populations and has been demonstrated in animals housed together under experimental conditions.[23] Routes of ferret-to-ferret transmission may include cannibalism and close contact activities such as den sharing, playing, fighting, mating, and feces sniffing.[23,27]

Although *M bovis* infection has been found in feral ferrets in New Zealand for decades, their host status is still subject to debate.[31–33] Are ferrets spillover hosts or maintenance hosts of *M bovis*? In a spillover host, intraspecies transmission of an infectious agent occurs; however, an outside source is required for disease to persist within the population.[33] Pathology and epidemiology suggest that, in most instances, ferrets are spillover hosts, and it is generally accepted that exposure to *M bovis*–infected possums determines the prevalence of disease in ferret populations.[5,6,31–33]

Although ferrets may chiefly be a spillover host of bovine tuberculosis, there is some evidence that tuberculosis can be maintained independently when ferret population densities are high.[3,31,32] The ferret's possible role as a maintenance host in bovine tuberculosis was first suggested in the early 1990s when in some cases sustained culling of possums did not achieve the desired reduction in tuberculosis among livestock.[23] Feral ferrets may serve as maintenance hosts in the semiarid regions with large rabbit colonies that do not support possum populations.[6,23,30,33] Therefore, the ferret's ability to serve as a potential source of infection for domestic livestock may vary with geography. Risk is usually low to moderate but may be high in specific areas.[33]

The controversy surrounding the host status of the feral ferret has created uncertainty as to whether active management of ferret populations is needed for the long-term control and eventual eradication of *M bovis* infection in livestock.[4,31] Culling of ferrets has been conducted and has been reported to reduce the incidence of tuberculosis in sympatric livestock, suggesting that ferret-to-livestock transmission of disease may occur.[30,32,34]

Bovine tuberculosis can be spread to cattle by a number of routes; however, inhalation is the most important method of transmission.[25] In what ways do ferrets excrete *M bovis* that could lead to infection in cattle? And do ferrets exhibit behavior that may enable cattle to encounter an infectious dose of *M bovis*? Ferrets are reported to frequently den in hay barns on cattle farms, so this may provide a route of transmission.[25,35] However, compared with possums, ferrets have relatively infrequent contact with cattle overall, making them a less likely source of infection,[25,34] and interactions between cattle and ferrets conducive to aerosol transmission are also extremely unlikely.[33] Tuberculous lung lesions are common in possums, which excrete *M bovis* in aerosols or discharges.[34] Tuberculous lesions in the ferret lung are rare.[34] Studies have also been conducted to evaluate and compare the response of livestock to ferrets and possums that were sedated so they would behave like terminally ill, tuberculous animals. Cattle, deer, and sheep showed interest in possums by sniffing and licking them, but they only briefly touched the ferrets and no licking or extended investigation was observed. In fact, cattle spent 7.7-fold more time in physical contact with possums compared to ferrets.[34]

Necropsy Findings in Ferrets with *M bovis* Infection

Tuberculous lesions in ferrets with *M bovis* infection are often difficult to discern,[3] and nearly one-third of infected ferrets may have no gross lesions at necropsy.[4,33] Many early changes in the lymph nodes such are enlargement are difficult to distinguish from the variable appearance of the normal lymph node, and caseous, necrotic foci are often so small as to be barely detectable with the naked eye.[4]

In a survey of 94 tuberculous feral ferrets with *M bovis* infection, a little over half (56.4%) had single-site lesions.[24] Nearly one-fourth (24.5%) of ferrets had multiple site infection and 19.1% had disseminated or generalized disease.[24] As seen with non–*M. bovis* infection in the ferret, initial lesions are most frequently associated with the gastrointestinal tract.[5] The lymph nodes that drain the gut, like the retropharyngeal and mesenteric or jejunal lymph nodes, are the most common site for infection.[24]

Primary infection of the lungs is rare.[4] In one survey, lesions involving the respiratory tract were found in only 2.9% of ferrets,[24] and none of the ferrets examined had extensive or advanced pulmonary lesions.[4] Nevertheless, the presence of lipid plaques, especially large ones, should alert the examiner to an increased possibility of *M bovis* infection. The presence of lipid plaques was found to be 2.4 times more likely in infected ferrets.[4,36] Lipid plaques are subpleural cream-colored plaques up to 6 mm in diameter that may be seen on the lung surface in infected and noninfected ferrets with endogenous lipid pneumonia.[4,36] These plaques contain mononuclear inflammatory cells, occasionally eosinophils, and in some instances cholesterol crystals.[4,36]

DIAGNOSIS OF MYCOBACTERIAL INFECTION IN FERRETS

Diagnosis of mycobacteriosis in ferrets may be based on cytology, identification of the organism via microbial and molecular methods, and pathology. Carefully examine lymph nodes for evidence of lymphadenitis. Necrotic foci have been reported in the retropharyngeal, mandibular, superficial axillary, caudal cervical, popliteal, inguinal, jejunal, or mesenteric and colonic lymph nodes.[4] Lesions are most frequently described in the retropharyngeal and mesenteric nodes.[4,24] Additional gross lesions will vary with the individual and the species of *Mycobacterium*; however, involvement of the stomach, intestines, spleen, liver, kidneys, lung, trachea, conjunctiva, middle and inner ear, brain, and/or skin have all been reported.[4,7–11,14–16,20,24] A more detailed description of some of the gross lesions observed with *M bovis* infection may be found above.

Histologically, the disease process in *M bovis* infection may not be as aggressive or tissue destructive in ferrets as in other species.[4] Lesions are typically necrotic and liquefactive with extensive macrophage infiltration, but fibrosis is relatively rare.[4,17] A prevalent histological finding in ferrets with *M bovis* infection is microscopic hepatic granulomas, although these lesions may be absent in early infections or in cases where disease is localized to peripheral lymph nodes.[4] Another common finding during evaluation of pulmonary tissue is entrapment of acid-fast organisms (AFOs) within lipid plaques on the lung's surface.[4,36]

AFOs may be identified within tissue using Ziehl-Neelsen staining. Within inflammatory foci, large numbers of AFOs are found within macrophages[7] (**Fig. 2**). Atypical mycobacterial infections are associated with sparse numbers of AFOs.[7] Suspect tissues, particularly lymph nodes, should be submitted for culture. *Mycobacterium* spp may also be identified by analysis of polymerase chain reaction from fresh biopsy material or from formalin-fixed paraffin-embedded tissue.[9]

Monitoring Wild Populations

In New Zealand, the majority of recent wildlife surveillance for bovine tuberculosis has relied on the use of ferrets as a sentinel species.[19,32] The prevalence of tuberculosis in possum populations is usually low (<2%).[37] To obtain some certainty that a population is free of infection requires examination of a high percentage of animals.[28] Surveys of ferret populations are much more cost-effective because ferrets have lower population densities, larger home ranges, and a higher prevalence of infection.[3,19,28]

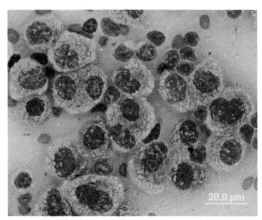

Fig. 2. Squash preparation of conjunctiva from an adult ferret (*Mustela putorius furo*) with *Mycobacterium genavense*. Large numbers of small, negative-staining bacilli may be seen within the macrophages of this DiffQuick-stained slide. (*Courtesy of* Dr Patricia Martin, Veterinary Pathology Diagnostic Services, University of Sydney, Sydney, Australia.)

Ferrets are monitored by trapping, necropsy, and bacterial culture of selected lymph nodes from animals with and without visible lesions.[3] Culture of pooled lymph node sample homogenates from up to 30 different ferrets has been found to be a sensitive method for detecting a significant proportion of *M bovis*–infected ferrets that would otherwise go undetected.[3]

ZOONOTIC POTENTIAL

The zoonotic potential of *Mycobacterium* spp has been well established,[1,21,38–40] although the specific risk of exposure to infected ferrets is unknown.[12] *M bovis* remains an important cause of human tuberculosis in developing nations but is relatively uncommon in most developed countries, including New Zealand, where *M bovis* infection is prevalent in feral ferrets.[1,38–40] Sixty human cases have been documented in New Zealand from 1985 to 1995.[1] Most of these infections occurred in elderly people and were probably acquired before introduction of milk pasteurization and herd testing in the 1940s and 1950s.[1] One interesting case report described *M bovis* infection following a ferret bite.[41] Reactivation of this dormant infection occurred 22 years after apparently successful treatment.[41] Veterinarians exposed to ferrets potentially infected with mycobacteriosis should follow standard preventive measures including appropriate hygiene and sanitation.

TREATMENT OPTIONS FOR FERRETS WITH MYCOBACTERIAL INFECTION

Euthanasia is often selected for ferrets with confirmed mycobacteriosis because of the perceived zoonotic potential of *Mycobacterium* spp and the organism's known resistance to the bacteriocidal mechanisms of antibiotics.[7,42] In human *M abscessus* respiratory infections, disease rarely resolves, and even with negative follow-up cultures, disease can recur when antibiotics are withdrawn.[43]

Nonetheless, treatments have been attempted and described in the literature for ferrets with mycobacteriosis, but scientific research is lacking. In one case report, disseminated *M abscessus* infection involving the respiratory tract was managed with clarithromycin (8 to 10 mg/kg orally twice daily for 3 months; Biaxin, Abbott).[8]

Treatment was considered successful based on cytology and culture results.[8] Another monotherapy that was deemed a failure involved the administration of rifampicin or rifampin (14 mg orally once daily for 6 weeks; Rifadin, Bedford Labs) to a 700-g ferret with disseminated *M genavense* infection involving the conjunctiva.[9] Two months after treatment was halted, the ferret presented in a moribund state. The animal was euthanized, but a full necropsy was not performed.[9]

In another case report, combination therapy for splenitis caused by *M celatum* consisting of enrofloxacin (5 mg/kg orally once daily; Baytril, Bayer), rifampicin (20 mg/kg orally twice daily), and azithromycin (10 mg/kg orally twice daily; Zithromax, Pfizer) resulted in initial clinical improvement. Although cytology was negative after 40 days, discontinuation of treatment was followed by rapid clinical deterioration and death.[10] Another regimen given for disseminated *M genavense* infection in a 1.2-kg ferret was rifampicin (30 mg orally once daily; Rifadin, Bedford Labs), clofazimine (12.5 mg orally once daily; Lamprene, Novartis), and clarithromycin (31.25 mg orally once daily; Biaxin, Abbott).[9] This combination therapy was reportedly successful, although both ferrets subsequently died as a result of other disease conditions, 4 and 10 months following initiation of therapy.[9]

VACCINATION

Studies have evaluated systemic and oral vaccination of ferrets with Bacille-Calmette-Guerin, or BCG, vaccine.[44,45] Although more work is needed, vaccination of feral ferrets in New Zealand may limit potential transmission of *M bovis* to livestock by reducing the severity and/or incidence of tuberculosis in wild populations.[44,45]

SUMMARY

The epidemiology of mycobacteriosis in the ferrets of New Zealand involves complex interactions between ferrets, possums, and livestock.[32] Investigators have shown that the ferret is highly susceptible only to *M bovis* infection and is more resistant to infection by other *Mycobacterium* spp.[4] The principal site of all mycobacterial infection in the ferret is the gastrointestinal tract.[33] Lymphadenitis is most commonly found in the lymph nodes that drain the intestinal tract.

REFERENCES

1. Baker MG, Lopez LD, Cannon MC, et al. Continuing *Mycobacterium bovis* transmission from animals to humans in New Zealand. Epidemiol Infect 2006;134:1068–73.
2. de Lisle GW, Crews K, de Zwart J, et al. *Mycobacterium bovis* infections in wild ferrets. New Zealand Vet J 1993;41:148–9.
3. de Lisle GW, Kawakami RP, Yates GF, et al. Isolation of *Mycobacterium bovis* and other mycobacterial species from ferrets and stoats. Vet Microbiol 2008;132(3-4): 402–7.
4. Lugton IW, Wobeser G, Morris RS, et al. Epidemiology of *Mycobacterium bovis* infection in feral ferrets (*Mustela furo*) in New Zealand: I. Pathology and diagnosis. N Z Vet J 1997;45:140–50.
5. Lugton IW, Wobeser G, Morris RS, et al. Epidemiology of *Mycobacterium bovis* infection in feral ferrets (*Mustela furo*) in New Zealand: II. Routes of infection and excretion. N Z Vet J 1997;45:151–7.
6. Ragg JR, Moller H, Waldrup KA. The prevalence of bovine tuberculosis (*Mycobacterium bovis*) infection in feral populations of cats (*Felis catus*), ferrets (*Mustela furo*), and stoats (*Mustela erminea*) in Otago and Southland, New Zealand: Implications for bovine tuberculosis transmission. N Z Vet J 1995;43:333–7.

7. Garner MM. "Osis", "itis", and virus: Differentiating mycobacteriosis, disseminated idiopathic myofasciitis, and systemic coronavirus in the domestic ferret. In: North American Veterinary Conference Proceedings. Orlando (FL), 2011.
8. Lunn JA, Martin P, Zaki S, et al. Pneumonia due to *Mycobacterium abscessus* in two domestic ferrets (*Mustela putorius furo*). Australian Vet J 2005;83:542–6.
9. Lucas J, Lucas A, Furber H, et al. *Mycobacterium genavense* infection in two aged ferrets with conjunctival lesions. Aust Vet J 2000;78:685–9.
10. Piseddu E, Trotta M, Tortoli E, et al. Detection and molecular characterization of *Mycobacterium celatum* as a cause of splenitis in a domestic ferret (*Mustela putorious furo*). J Comp Pathol 2011;144:214–8.
11. Schultheiss P, Dolginow S. Granulomatous enteritis caused by *Mycobacterium avium* in a ferret. J Am Vet Med Assoc 1994;204:1217–8.
12. Fox JG. Bacterial and mycoplasmal diseases. In: Fox JG, editor. Biology and diseases of the Ferret, 2nd edition. Baltimore (MD): Williams & Wilkins; 1998. p. 321–54.
13. Emmanuel FX, Seagar AL, Doig C, et al. Human and animal infections with *Mycobacterium microti*, Scotland. Emerg Infect Dis 2007;13:1924–7.
14. Ludwig E. Risk for *Mycobacterium celatum* infection from ferret. Emerg Infect Dis 2011;17:553–5.
15. Valheim M, Djønne B, Heiene R, et al. Disseminated *Mycobacterium celatum* (type 3) infection in a domestic ferret (*Mustela putorious furo*). Vet Pathol 2001;38:460–3.
16. van Soolingen D, van der Zanden AGB, de Hass PEW, et al. Diagnosis of *Mycobacterium microti* infections among humans by using novel genetic markers. J Clin Microbiol 1998;36:1840–5.
17. Cross ML, Labes RE, Mackintosh CG. Oral infection of ferrets with virulent *Mycobacterium bovis* or *Mycobacterium avium*: susceptibility, pathogenesis and immune response. J Comp Pathol 2000;123:15–21.
18. Bryant JL, Hanner TL, Fultz DG, et al. A chronic granulomatous intestinal disease in ferrets caused by an acid-fast organism morphologically similar to *Mycobacterium paratuberculosis*. Lab Anim Sci 1998;38:498–9.
19. de Lisle GW, Yates GF, Cavaignac SM, et al. *Mycobacterium avium* subsp. *paratuberculosis* in feral ferrets — a potential reservoir of Johne's disease. In: Proceedings of the Seventh International Colloquium on Paratuberculosis. Bilbao (Spain), 2002. p. 361–2.
20. Viallier J, Vialler G, Prave M, et al. Place de *Mycobacterium avium* dans l'epidemiolgies mycobacterienne actuelle chez les animaux domestiques et sauvages. Sci Vet Med Comp 1983;85:103–9.
21. Orcau A, Caylà JA, Martínez JA. Present epidemiology of tuberculosis. Prevention and control programs. Enferm Infecc Microbiol Clin 2011;29(Suppl 1):2–7.
22. Saunders GK, Thomsen BV. Lymphoma and *Mycobacterium avium* infection in a ferret (*Mustela putorius furo*). J Vet Diagn 2006;18:513–5.
23. Qureshi T, Labes RE, Lambeth M, et al. Transmission of *Mycobacterium bovis* from experimentally infected ferrets to non-infected ferrets (*Mustela furo*). N Z Vet J 2000;48:99–104.
24. Ragg JR, Waldrup KA, Moller H. The distribution of gross lesions of tuberculosis caused by *Mycobacterium bovis* in feral ferrets (*Mustela furo*) from Otago, New Zealand. N Z Vet J 1995;43:338–41.
25. Phillips CJC, Foster CRW, Morris PA, et al. The transmission of *Mycobacterium bovis* infection to cattle. Res Vet Sci 2003;74:1–15.
26. Paterson BM, Morris RS. Interactions between beef cattle and simulated tuberculous possums on pasture. N Z Vet J 1995;43:289–93.

27. Ragg JR, Mackintosh CG, Moller H. The scavenging behaviour of ferrets (*Mustela furo*), feral cats (*Felis domesticus*), possums (*Trichosurus vulpecula*), hedgehogs (*Erinaceus europaeus*) and harrier hawks (*Circus approximans*) on pastoral farmland in New Zealand: Implications for bovine tuberculosis transmission. N Z Vet J 2000; 48:166–75.

28. de Lisle GW, Yates GF, Caley P, et al. Surveillance of wildlife for *Mycobacterium bovis* infection using culture of pooled tissue samples from ferrets (*Mustela furo*). N Z Vet J 2004;53:14–8.

29. Ragg JR, Waldrup KA, Moller H. Bovine tuberculosis infections of ferrets, stoats and feral cats in Otago, New Zealand. In: Deer Branch Course No. 11. Queenstown: Deer Branch of the New Zealand Veterinary Association; 1994. p. 114–26.

30. Caley P. Broad-scale possum and ferret correlates of macroscopic *Mycobacterium bovis* infection in feral ferret populations. N Z Vet J 1998;46:157–62.

31. Caley P, Hone J, Cowan PE. The relationship between prevalence of *Mycobacterium bovis* infection in feral ferrets and possum abundance. N Z Vet J 2001;49:195–200.

32. Ryan TJ, Livingstone PG, Ramsey DSL, et al. Advances in understanding disease epidemiology and implications for control and eradication of tuberculosis in livestock: The experience from New Zealand. Vet Microbiol 2006;112:211–9.

33. Corner LAL. The role of wild animal populations in the epidemiology of tuberculosis in domestic animals: How to assess the risk. Vet Microbiol 2006;112:303–12.

34. Sauter CM, Morris RS. Behavioural studies on the potential for direct transmission of tuberculosis from feral ferrets (*Mustela furo*) and possums (*Trichosurus vulpecula*) to farmed livestock. N Z Vet J 1995;43:294–300.

35. Ragg JR. The denning behaviour of feral ferrets (*Mustela furo*) in a pastoral habitat, South Island, New Zealand. J Zool 1998;246:471–7.

36. Symmers WStC, Thomson APD, Iland C. Observations on tuberculosis in the ferret (*Mustela furo*). J Comp Pathol 1953;63:20–31.

37. Pfeiffer DU, Hickling GJ, Morris RS, et al. The epidemiology of *Mycobacterium bovis* infection in brushtail possums (*Trichosurus vulpecula* Kerr) in the Hauhaungaroa Ranges, New Zealand. N Z Vet J 1995;43:272–80.

38. Cosivi O, Grange JM, Daborn CJ, et al. Zoonotic tuberculosis due to *Mycobacterium bovis* in developing countries. Emerg Infect Dis 1998;4:59–70.

39. Grange JM. *Mycobacterium bovis* infection in human beings. Tuberculosis (Edinb) 2001;81:71–7.

40. Michel AL, Muller B, van Helden PD. *Mycobacterium bovis* at the animal-human interface: a problem, or not? Vet Microbiol 2010;140:371–81.

41. Jones JW. Recurrent *Mycobacterium bovis* infection following a ferret bite. J Infect 1993;26:225–6.

42. Cross ML, Aldwell FE, Griffin JFT, et al. Intracellular survival of virulent *Mycobacterium bovis* and *M bovis* BCG in ferret macrophages. Vet Microbiol 1999;66:235–43.

43. Holland SM. Nontuberculous mycobacteria. Am J Med Sci 2001;321:49–55.

44. Cross ML, Labes RE, Griffin JFT, et al. Systemic but not intra-intestinal vaccination with BCG reduces the severity of tuberculosis in ferrets (*Mustela furo*). Int J Tuberc Lung Dis 2000;4:473–80.

45. Qureshi T, Labes RE, Cross ML, et al. Partial protection against oral challenge with Mycobacterium bovis in ferrets (Mustela furo) following oral vaccination with BCG. Int J Tuberc Lung Dis 1999;3:1025–33.

Index

Note: Page numbers of article titles are in **boldface** type.

A

Abscesses. See *Skin lesions.*
Acid-fast bacillus (AFB) staining, for mycobacteria, 1, 3, 72, 76
    in animal models, 27, 29–30, 33–35
    in birds, 41, 43–45, 48–51, 60
    in ferrets, 122
    in rabbits, 87
    in reptiles, 102, 105, 107–109
    in rodents, 88–89
    respiratory samples and, 77
AFB. See *Acid-fast bacillus (AFB) staining.*
Air sacs, avian mycobacteriosis effect on, 44–45, 47, 51
    clinical signs of, 72
Airway structures, mycobacteriosis effect on, in birds, 47, 49
    in ferrets, 122
Albumin level, mycobacteriosis effect on, 74, 87
Alligators, mycobacteriosis in, 102–104
Amikacin, for mycobacteriosis, 62, 105
Amino acid sequencing, 3
Aminoglycosides, for avian mycobacteriosis, 60–62
Aminosalicylic acid (PAS), for avian mycobacteriosis, 60, 62
Amphibian mycobacteriosis, **113–119**
   clinical aspects of, 28–30
   clinical signs and syndromes of, 72, 115–116
   diagnosis of, 116
   Mycobacterium species detected in, 113–115
   pathogenesis of, 115
   summary overview of, 113, 118
   treatment of, 117
   zoonotic considerations of, 117
Amyloidosis, with avian mycobacteriosis, 46–47
Anemia, with mycobacteriosis, in birds, 42, 74
    in rabbits, 87
Animal models, of mycobacteriosis, **25–40**. See also *specific animal.*
   amphibians as, 28–30
   ferrets as, 34–35
   fish as, 27–28
   rabbits as, 34
   reptiles as, 30–33, 107–108
   rodents as, 33–34
   summary overview of, 25–26, 35–36
   zoonotic potential in, 26, 59

Vet Clin Exot Anim 15 (2012) 131–153
doi:10.1016/S1094-9194(11)00092-2
1094-9194/12/$ – see front matter © 2012 Elsevier Inc. All rights reserved.

Moving?

Make sure your subscription moves with you!

To notify us of your new address, find your **Clinics Account Number** (located on your mailing label above your name), and contact customer service at:

Email: journalscustomerservice-usa@elsevier.com

800-654-2452 (subscribers in the U.S. & Canada)
314-447-8871 (subscribers outside of the U.S. & Canada)

Fax number: 314-447-8029

**Elsevier Health Sciences Division
Subscription Customer Service
3251 Riverport Lane
Maryland Heights, MO 63043**

*To ensure uninterrupted delivery of your subscription, please notify us at least 4 weeks in advance of move.

Printed and bound by CPI Group (UK) Ltd, Croydon, CR0 4YY

03/10/2024

01040446-0014